MY FIRST MRCP BOOK

PUBLISHED BY THE REMEDICA GROUP

Remedica Publishing Ltd, 32–38 Osnaburgh Street, London, NW1 3ND, UK
Remedica Inc, Tri-State International Center, Building 25, Suite 150, Lincolnshire, IL 60069, USA

E-mail: books@remedica.com
www.remedica.com

Publisher: Andrew Ward
In-house editor: Thomas Moberly

ISBN 1 901346 5 01

British Library Cataloguing-in Publication Data
A catalogue record for this book is available from the British Library

MY FIRST MRCP BOOK

HUGH MONTGOMERY
Rayne Institute
UCL Hospitals
London
UK

NEIL GOLDSACK
Kent and Canterbury Hospital
Kent
UK

RICHARD MARSHALL
Centre for Respiratory Research
UCL Hospitals
London
UK

WITH ADDITIONAL CONTRIBUTIONS FROM:
HOUMAN ASHRAFIAN
Hammersmith Hospital
London
UK

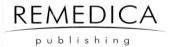

REMEDICA
publishing

CONTENTS

1   The strategy   1

2   Nervous ticks on the list   17

3   Pants   49

4   Metabollocks   65

5   Have a heart...   121

6   Skinny dips   133

7   Gastrointestinal tracts   145

8   A bloody hell   179

9   Taking the p**s   209

10 Sex!   223

11 Mopping up   231

12 More on the eponymous conditions in the MRCP examination   275

13 Those infamous lists again   279

INTRODUCTION

Gaining membership of the Royal College of Physicians (MRCP) is, in many ways, like a first sexual experience: most, even modestly attractive, people tend to get around to it in the end (think surgeons); peer pressure makes many try when they aren't quite ready; those that haven't are unsure what it's like; those who plan to have often been fed a variety of myths about how to; first attempts are often embarrassing and short-lived; and those who have been successful always claim to have sweated over it for hours, obtaining high scores first time. The very elderly can't remember how and some don't even know if they ever did.

On the other hand, MRCP is generally a more expensive business by far.

This book hopes to dispel some of the myths and to teach you all you need to know in an enjoyable and informative way. It is, if you will, 'The joy of membership' – a hands-on guide. We recognise, of course, that the MRCP exam format changes. However, the basic knowledge required does not, and nor has the approach which can be used. This book, therefore, remains truly 'your first MRCP Book'. Its use is not restricted, however: all students of medicine (including those who practice!) will hone diagnostic skills.

Whatever. Too much foreplay.

Starting from page 1, we shall teach you in a step-by-step fashion, in the privacy of your own room. By the time you reach the end, we hope that you will have all the skills you need. However, we would still advise you to go and buy other books in the field and practice what you have learned.

We hope that this book will give pleasure, as much to the student as to the more qualified reader and, whoever you are, we hope that you will enjoy your lessons. But remember – don't leave your room smiling. Maintain the myth of the tortured youth.

How to use this book

This book is **not** just another compilation of questions, and you should not treat it as such. It is a complete and structured course. If you start on page 1 and work steadily through to the end, you will have learned not just the facts you need but a strategy of attack. Dipping into the book randomly in search of questions will, we promise, be a pretty unrewarding business.

We have put a great deal of time and effort into the preparation of this book.

- We have assumed reasonable background knowledge. If you hit upon a diagnosis about which you remember little, then look it up elsewhere.

- We have emphasised the subject matter that commonly appears in the examination.

- We are, however, aware that it may be difficult for you to accumulate adequate information on some of the more obscure topics and we have attended to these in more detail. Short texts on these subjects are given where knowledge may be thin.

- We have structured it so that you build on knowledge. You will need facts learned early in the book to be able to answer questions later on.

We have also tried to use a little sensible educational theory. We all learn in different ways and sticking to one way is tedious, so we have provided a variety of tools: historical vignettes, mnemonics, pictures, poems, puzzles, tables, and equations. Intermittently, you will come across a puzzle, joke, or other form of amusement. Please do not rush over these – they are designed to reinforce facts you have already learned. They are also spaced so as to 'give your brain a rest' between more intensive bouts of cramming.

Once you have read and learned, then every other book on the market becomes a practice ground for you. We would strongly encourage you to buy a generous selection of these, as ultimately there is no substitute for practice.

So off you go. Slow and steady from start to finish.

Do learn.

And, please, do enjoy too.

THE STRATEGY

Are you sitting comfortably? Then let us
begin. Start by having a go at this first
question. Don't look anything up – just
make a stab at it. All will be revealed when
you turn the page.

Q1

A 12-year-old girl of Nigerian origin lives with her parents and grandparents. She has a 5-year-old brother who has recently suffered an acute coryzal illness. Her mother is a primary school teacher, while her father is in the diplomatic service; the family move biannually to different countries. The family returned to the UK from Peru only 3 months ago, having spent their final month visiting ancient Inca tombs. The girl presents to her local Accident and Emergency Department with a 10-day history of fever and general malaise. Twenty days before her presentation she had received a 1-week course of antibiotics from her GP for a throat infection. The family kitten (an adopted and unvaccinated stray that was smuggled through customs) died of an unknown infection 3 weeks earlier. In addition to her fever, she complains of several days' pain and swelling in both wrists, her left knee and right ankle, which she attributes to a recent hockey training session. Her mother can remember no past history of joint problems.

ON EXAMINATION

- T = 39.4°C
- Pulse = 98 beats/min regular
- BP = 105/70 mmHg
- JVP not elevated
- Mouth clear
- No rashes or LAN
- Chest clear
- HS 1 + 2 + soft ESM left sternal edge
- Abdomen soft, no HSM
- Painful, hot and swollen wrists, knee and ankle (see above)

INVESTIGATIONS

- Hb = 10.5 g/l
- U & E = normal
- Urinalysis:
  normal dipstick
  no casts/cells
  negative cultures
- MCV = 89 fl
- Bilirubin = 8 μmol/l
- WCC = 13 x 10^9/l
- Neutrophils = 85%
- Platelets = 450 x 10^9/l
- ESR = 130 mm in first hour
- AST = 70 IU/l
- CRP = 76 mg/l
- Chest X-ray = normal
- ECG = sinus rhythm (see **Figure 1**), PR interval 0.3 s, QRS 0.12 s, QT 0.4 s, normal axis

AST: aspartate aminotransferase; BP: blood pressure; CRP: C-reactive protein; ECG: electrocardiogram; ESM: ejection systolic murmur; ESR: erythrocyte sedimentation rate; Hb: haemoglobin; HS: heart sounds; HSM: hepatosplenomegaly; JVP: jugular venous pulse; LAN: lymphadenopathy; MCV: mean corpuscular volume; T: temperature; U & E: urinalysis and electrolytes; WCC: white cell count.

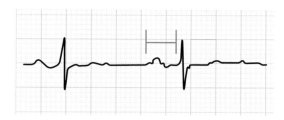

Figure 1. ECG in sinus rhythm.

a) **What is the most likely diagnosis?**
   i)   polyarticular Still's disease
   ii)   acute rheumatic fever
   iii) coccidioidomycosis
   iv)   toxocariasis
   v)   toxoplasmosis

b) **Which investigation will confirm your diagnosis?**
   i)   autoantibody screen
   ii)   haemoglobin electrophoresis
   iii) rheumatoid factor
   iv)   blood cultures
   v)   acute and convalescent serum antistreptolysin O (ASO) titres
   vi)   left knee aspiration, microscopy and culture
   vii) toxoplasmosis serology
   viii) toxocariasis serology

c) **What is the appropriate management? Select three of the following:**
   i)   corticosteroid therapy
   ii)   acetylsalicylate
   iii) bed rest
   iv)   penicillamine
   v)   physiotherapy
   vi)   family screening and counselling
   vii) opiate analgesia
   viii) appropriate antibiotic therapy
   ix)   fluconazole or amphotericin
   x)   trimethoprim

The first stage in answering a 'grey case', such as this, is to recognise the examiners' tactics. Invariably, they have marred the clarity of any story with 'smoke and mirrors' – extraneous facts that just cause confusion. Some are in there as meaningless bulk, while others are there as malicious red herrings. But then again, this pretty much emulates real life!

The key, then, is to positively ignore the waffle, and *seek out only those features of the examination and investigations that you know are always pathological*. Is the fact that the cat died always pathological for the patient? No. Is the fact that she is Nigerian? No. Is the fact that they were recently in Peru? No! And Inca graves? Nonsense! These factors might later be helpful in confirming a diagnosis, but not making it: at the moment they are nothing more than white smoke. Or tear gas. So what *are* the findings which are always pathological? They are:

- fever
- polyarthropathy
- normochromic normocytic anaemia
- elevated WCC with leucocytosis
- elevated AST
- elevated ESR and CRP
- prolonged PR interval

Of these, some are quite nonspecific, such as fever. In fact, you can dismiss most of these findings as nonspecific. Fever, elevated ESR, raised CRP, raised white cell count... Hmmm. She is suffering an acute inflammatory condition. Well, no s**t, Sherlock! So now identify which of these has only a limited list of potential causes and hone in on these. Finally, write down the list of causes for each abnormal feature you have identified.

In this case, the features that are always abnormal and that have a limited list of causes are *polyarthropathy* and *first-degree heart block*.

The causes of polyarthropathy are principally rheumatological, infectious, and haematological...

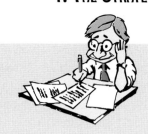

CAUSES OF POLYARTHRALGIA

Joint attacks are done by three –
RA, Still's, and HSP
Pyrophosphate, SLE
And seronegativity

Parvo, clap, group A, TB,
Germans, chicken pox, Hep B
Spread by ticks (and not by fleas)
Is the dreaded Lyme disease

Sarcoid, i/c, SBE
Hepatitis A,B,C
Coming over sickle-y
With widespread malignancy

FMF and Behçet's do
Chronic hepatitis, too
Crohn's and Whipple's, never fear!
UC shall bring up 'the rear'!

Behçet's: Behçet's syndrome; clap: gonorrhoea; Crohn's: Crohn's disease; FMF: familial Mediterranean fever; Germans: German measles (rubella); group A: group A beta-haemolytic *Streptococcus*; Hep: hepatitis; HIV: human immunodeficiency virus; HSP: Henoch–Schönlein purpura; Parvo: parvovirus; RA: rheumatoid arthritis; SBE: subacute bacterial endocarditis; SLE: systemic lupus erythematosus; Still's: Still's disease; TB: tuberculosis; UC: ulcerative colitis; Whipple's: Whipple's disease

Remember that seronegative joint inflammation may be due to osteoarthritis, as well as reactive arthritis (Reiter's syndrome), Poncet's (tuberculous rheumatism), ankylosing spondylitis, ulcerative colitis, and Crohn's disease. Haemochromatosis is an example of a metabolic cause, and leukaemia in children is an example of a malignant cause, often of monoarthritis but also polyarthritis. In addition, remember the haematological causes, such as sickle cell disease, which can give rise to hand-and-foot syndrome. In addition, septic polyarthritis can occur when joints are seeded with organisms such as *Neisseria gonorrheae* or *Staphylococcus*.

How many of these are associated with a long PR interval? You probably do not even have to remember a list, as three come almost immediately to mind: acute rheumatic fever, sarcoidosis, and Lyme disease. It is likely to be one of these three. Now you return to the history. It is unlikely to be Lyme disease as she has not been wandering around the New Forest. She does not have the characteristic erythema nodosum or bilateral hilar lymphadenopathy of sarcoidosis. She has, however, had a recent sore throat. Which fits best? Evidently, acute rheumatic fever, and this is where you put your money.

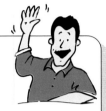

A1   **a) Diagnosis**
Acute rheumatic fever

b) Investigation
Acute and convalescent ASO titres

c) Management
Acetylsalicylate
Bed rest
Physiotherapy

Did you know the causes of a long PR interval? If not come up with a list and a way to remember them. Jot them down here.

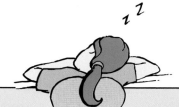

REVISION ZONE

Revised Duckett-Jones criteria for acute rheumatic fever

MAJOR	Pancarditis
	Polyarthropathy
	Sydenham's chorea
	Erythema marginatum
	Subcutaneous nodules (Aschoff nodules)
MINOR	Prolonged PR interval
	Arthralgia (not applicable if polyarthropathy is used as a major criterion)
	Elevated ESR/CRP
	Past rheumatic fever
	Leucocytosis

The diagnosis of acute rheumatic fever rests on evidence of a recent streptococcal infection (acute and convalescent ASO titres; positive throat cultures for group A *Streptococcus*; streptococcal antibodies) and at least:

two MAJOR criteria

or one MAJOR and at least two MINOR criteria

The patient in the case history has one major and three minor criteria: polyarthropathy + prolonged PR interval, elevated ESR/CRP, and leucocytosis

Now, check that you have learnt the causes of a long PR interval, the causes of polyarthropathy, and the diagnostic criteria for rheumatic fever. When you are absolutely confident that you can write out the lists, you may move on!

A QUICK JOKE

Talking of PRs, the tale is told of a rather quick-witted but lazy house surgeon. After a long night on the beers, he had clerked a patient in somewhat of a rush, and was now presenting him on the ward round. "Abdomen soft and nontender", he said. "No LK2S or nodes. PR NAD." The professor went puce. "PR NAD?" he howled. "NAD? This man has had an abdomino-perineal resection! What do you mean, PR NAD?" The house officer looked the professor straight in the eye. "No anus detected", he replied.

Q2 A 14-year-old girl presented to her local Accident and Emergency Department with a 10-day history of fever and malaise, which have prevented her going to school. She is of European origin and lives with her parents and her 5-year-old brother who has been in complete remission from acute lymphoblastic leukaemia (ALL) for 1 year. Her mother is a primary school teacher while her father is in the diplomatic service, necessitating the family to make biannual moves abroad. They now live near the 'Elaphos Priory' outside Southampton. Ten days before the onset of her symptoms, her GP gave her a 1-week course of antibiotics for a throat infection. In addition to her fever, she complains of several days' pain and swelling in both wrists, her left knee and right ankle. She mentions an annular rash on her right arm, which she noticed a few weeks ago, but which now appears to be fading.

ON EXAMINATION

- T = 39°C
- Pulse = 98 beats/min regular
- BP = 105/70 mmHg
- JVP not elevated
- Mouth clear
- No LAN
- Chest clear
- HS 1 + 2 + soft ESM left sternal edge
- Abdomen soft, no HSM
- Painful, hot and swollen wrists, left knee and right ankle
- Annular erythema on right arm

INVESTIGATIONS

- Hb = 12 g/l
- U & E = normal
- Urinalysis:
  normal dipstick
  no casts/cells
  negative cultures
- MCV = 89 fl
- Bilirubin = 8 μmol/l
- WCC = 13 x 10^9/l
- Neutrophils = 85%
- Platelets = 450 x 10^9/l
- ESR = 130 mm in first hour
- AST = 45 IU/l
- CRP = 76 mg/l
- Chest X-ray = normal
- ECG = sinus rhythm, PR interval 0.3 s, QRS 0.12 s, QT 0.4 s, normal axis

AST: aspartate aminotransferase; BP: blood pressure; CRP: C-reactive protein; ECG: electrocardiogram; ESM: ejection systolic murmur; ESR: erythrocyte sedimentation rate; Hb: haemoglobin; HS: heart sounds; HSM: hepatosplenomegaly; JVP: jugular venous pulse; LAN: lymphadenopathy; MCV: mean corpuscular volume; T: temperature; U & E: urinalysis and electrolytes; WCC: white cell count.

a) What is the most likely diagnosis?

i) polyarticular Still's disease
ii) acute rheumatic fever
iii) hand-and-foot syndrome of sickle cell disease
iv) Lyme disease

b) Which one investigation will confirm your diagnosis?

i) antinuclear antibody (ANA) and autoantibody screen
ii) haemoglobin electrophoresis
iii) rheumatoid factor
iv) blood cultures
v) acute and convalescent serum ASO titres
vi) left knee aspiration, microscopy, and culture
vii) anti-*Borrelia burgdorferi* IgM antibodies

c) What is the appropriate management? Select three of the following:

i) corticosteroid therapy
ii) nonsteroidal antiinflammatories (NSAIDs)
iii) bed rest
iv) intravenous ceftriaxone
v) penicillamine
vi) physiotherapy
vii) opiate analgesia

The case history here is similar to the previous one and similar lists for polyarthropathy and a prolonged PR interval can be used to aid with the diagnosis. As before, the history is important in determining the most likely diagnosis and allows a diagnosis different to the first case to be reached. It is the *annular* rash that is the clue, and is designed to suggest erythema chronicum migrans rather than erythema marginatum, making Lyme disease the most likely diagnosis.

Bonus points for any Greek scholars: *elaphos* is Greek for 'deer'. Out of interest (but don't bother to learn it!), Lyme disease is tick-transmitted by *Ixodes dammini* in the USA, *I. ricinus* in Europe and *I. parascapularis* in Asia. Lyme disease was first described in 1977 in Old Lyme, Connecticut, USA.

A2 a) **Diagnosis**
Lyme disease

b) **Investigation**
Detection of antibody to *B. burgdorferi* in serum

c) **Management**
Intravenous ceftriaxone (or cefotaxime)
Salicylate analgesia
Physiotherapy

Note that in the presence of the characteristic rash and fever alone, i.e. without any of the joint/cardiological/neurological complications, oral tetracycline (doxycycline) or penicillin is sufficient. Note the similarities to syphilis, another spirochaetal disease.

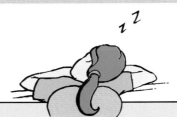

REVISION ZONE: LYME DISEASE

There are three main phases:

1) EARLY LOCALISED DISEASE (within days)
Erythema chronicum migrans
Associated symptoms: malaise, fever, arthralgia, stiff neck

2) EARLY DISSEMINATED DISEASE (within weeks)
Cardiological: myocarditis or pancarditis with conduction disturbances
Neurological: lymphocytic meningitis, encephalitis, cranial nerve palsies, Bannwarth's syndrome, mononeuritis
Musculoskeletal: polyarthritis
Renal: microhaematuria
Hepatic: hepatitis
Ocular: iritis, conjunctivitis
Dermatological: erythema nodosum
Lymphadenopathy

3) LATE DISSEMINATED DISEASE (within months to years)
Musculoskeletal: migratory polyarthritis
Neurological: chronic neuroborreliosis, dementia
Dermatological: acrodermatitis chronic atrophicans *(Borrelia afzelii)*

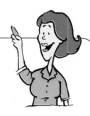

Q3 A 43-year-old woman presents with headaches. Until 3 years ago she was an airline stewardess, but now works at a ticket desk at the airport. She is married with three children, all of whom are in good health. She was well until 2 weeks ago when she developed severe headaches that started waking her up in the early hours of the morning. The headaches are pounding in nature, characteristically starting behind her right eye and she says that her husband mentioned that her eye had gone red on one occasion. She has also noticed that the headache is associated with a feeling of having a blocked nose and this tends to occur with a runny eye. Her past medical history is unremarkable. She has suffered from irritable bowel in the past, but this has settled over the last 6 years. She is not taking any medication.

ON EXAMINATION	INVESTIGATIONS
• Unremarkable	• CT scan of the head: NAD

CT: computed tomography; NAD: no abnormality detected.

a) What is the most likely diagnosis?

Whoops. The answer here is hard to tease out, as there are no clear associated lists, and this is where the 'list' method breaks down. This is one of those questions that you either recognise as a 'classic textbook description', or you haven't a clue and, therefore, get no marks. Not at all fair, although the membership examination does unfortunately love questions like this. However, there aren't that many of them, and we'll try to cover most of them as we go along. Shy–Drager syndrome is a classic and so too is phenytoin overdose; a typical example is of a recurrently ataxic child with an epileptic grandma – the damn kid has been eating her pills.

You can usually tell that a question is one of the 'classics' due to the lack of differentiating signs associated with a 'list'. Here, the history of severe headaches with nasal stuffiness and runny eyes should alert you to an odd diagnosis.

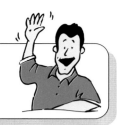

A3 a) Diagnosis
Migrainous neuralgia

ADDITIONAL BITS: THE BULLS**T BOX AND THE SURGICAL SIEVE

Some features in the history can give you clues. Traditionally, the examiners have been very keen to stereotype certain occupations with certain diseases, so below is a list of these.

BULLS**T BOX

PROFESSION	DISEASE
Health care professionals	Factitious illnesses (e.g. hypoglycaemia due to recurrent insulin administration)
Farmers	Farmer's lung
Scientists	Weil's disease or rat allergies
Barman/civil servant	Alcoholism
Travelling businessmen/bachelors	Sexually transmitted diseases

We apologise to these professions, but it is honestly not our fault. In fact, some traditional stereotypes appear in the examinations, but are too defamatory to print in this book. Keep your eyes open, and prepare your own list! And once you have it, keep it to yourself. For remember the two most important rules in life:

1) DON'T TELL EVERYONE EVERYTHING YOU KNOW

2)

Occasionally, your mind might go blank when faced with a question. You can spot the obvious pathology, but cannot remember the appropriate list. Under such circumstances, you need to make up your own list 'on the hoof'. We have a strategy for this, involving the mnemonic 'TIE HIM IN': trauma, infection, endocrine, haematological, iatrogenic, metabolic, idiopathic, neoplastic. For almost all of these, there is a subdivision as follows:

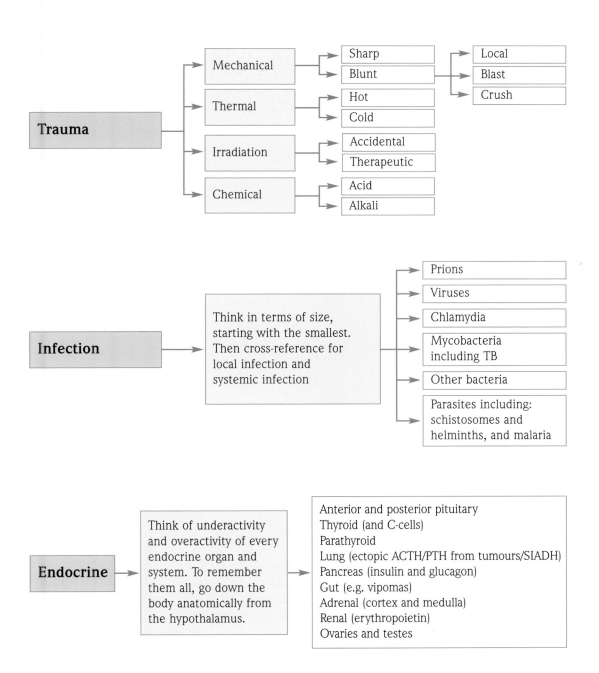

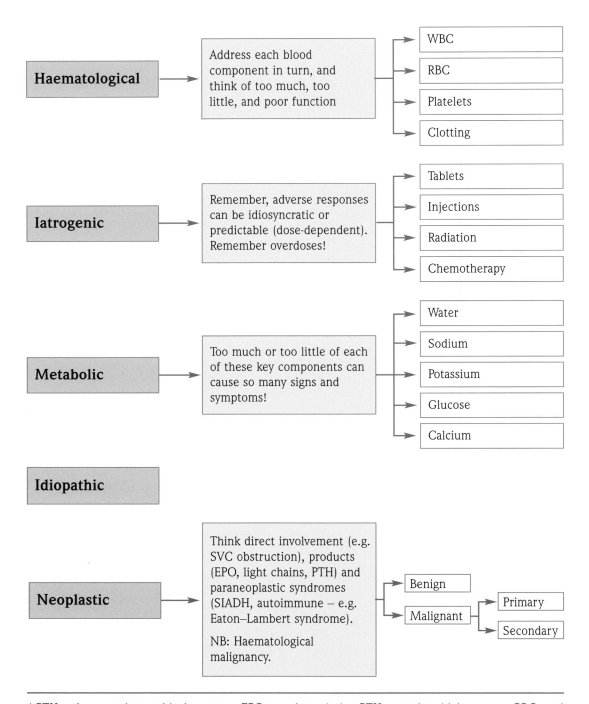

ACTH: adrenocorticotrophic hormone; EPO: erythropoietin; PTH: parathyroid hormone; RBC: red blood cell; SIADH: syndrome of inappropriate antidiuretic hormone; SVC: superior vena cava; TB: tuberculosis; WBC: white blood cell

CROSS-CHECKS

Once you have gone through this sieve, run through a few final cross-checks. Have you checked:

- each system in turn: respiratory, central nervous system, etc.
- occupational, tropical, and autoimmune diseases
- those diseases peculiar to the young or old
- the usual suspects (SLE, sarcoidosis, amyloidosis, tuberculosis)

If nothing on your list seems to fit, then think:

- overdose? (Has the patient been eating grandma's phenytoin?)
- is this a 'syndrome' I should recognise?

Always remember intoxication and drugs – you can be sure that the patient and examiners will lay you traps.

SUMMARY

From these questions, you should be able to see how to tackle the membership paper. These are the same rules that we use when making a diagnosis on the wards or in the clinic. The plan is simple:

1) Ignore the 'white smoke' and write down all the findings that are *always abnormal*

2) From these findings, select those for which there are a *limited list* of potential causes

3) Write down the list of causes for each finding. Don't worry – we shall be teaching you these as we go along. You have already learnt two

4) Look at the lists you have written down. The correct diagnosis must appear on all the lists. If there is only one overlapping factor, then this is the diagnosis you seek

5) If there is more than one diagnosis that appears on all your lists, then go through factors that might *exclude* some diagnoses

6) Look at those you have left. From the information you have available, select the diagnosis that fits best, and run with this one

If there seem to be no useful lists, then it is likely that this is one of the 'you either recognise it or you don't' questions. There is not much of a strategy to adopt here. However, we will try to cover most of the 'classic cases' as we go along.

Rather than going through lists in random order, we shall try to approach them in groupings by system or symptom. You will find that lists appear again and again; this is to help you learn by repetition. We have also tried to vary the way in which you can learn a list; some are alphabetical, some equations, some mnemonics, some acronyms, and some appear as pictures or verse. Please do not feel constrained by the way lists are presented – feel free to find a way of your own to remember them.

Good luck and enjoy. Remember, like other books in the 'Joys of ...' series, you can work on this alone, or even better with friends, anytime and anywhere!

QUIZ SPOT!

CRITERIA CONNECTIONS

Connect the Duckett-Jones Criteria to the right class: major criteria or minor criteria. Which ones are missing and how many criteria are needed to make the diagnosis of Rheumatic Fever (answers on page 185)?

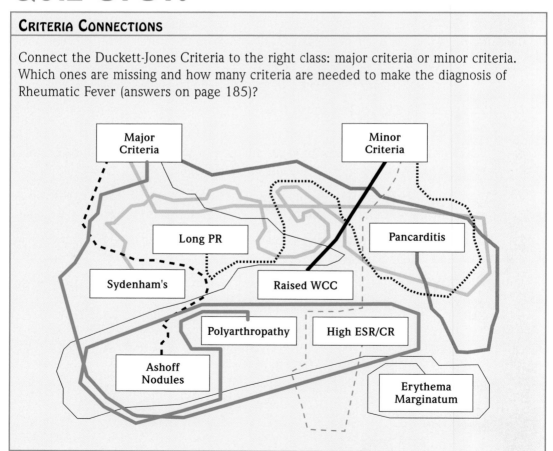

2

NERVOUS TICKS ON THE LIST

NEUROLOGICAL MRCP LISTS

CAUSES OF INTRACRANIAL CALCIFICATION

Tumours	Glioma (astrocytoma, oligodendroglioma), meningioma, craniopharyngioma (90% in children), ependymoma, pinealoma, teratoma, chordoma, dermoid, cholesteatoma. Lipomas are usually midline and have typical curved bands of calcification
Vascular	Atheroma, aneurysm, angioma, sub-dural haematoma, and intracerebral haematoma
Infection and infestation (often multiple)	Tuberculosis (basal meninges), toxoplasmosis (paraventricular), cytomegalovirus, cysticercosis (usually supratentorial), pyogenic abscess, hydatid, and *Paragonimus westermani*
Miscellaneous	Phakomatosis: tuberous sclerosis, Sturge–Weber syndrome (characterised by tram lines), von Hippel–Lindau syndrome, neurofibromatosis types 1 and 2, and Gorlin's syndrome. Renal failure plus dialysis
Basal ganglia	Birth anoxia (idiopathic (most common) bilateral and symmetrical), radiation, mitochondrial diseases, Fahr's disease, hypoparathyroidism, pseudohypoparathyroidism, and infarction

Q4 A 72-year-old man presents complaining that he has had to give up smoking against his will. Painters have been redecorating his flat for some weeks. He has been effectively housebound and feels he has been continually exposed to the fumes. His smoker's cough has worsened and precipitated his cigarette abstinence. His GP has prescribed erythromycin and amoxycillin for what has appeared to be an almost constant cough. He has taken arrowroot as a homeopathic remedy. He has found it increasingly difficult to handle his cigarettes and matches during this period. He says that his hand is weak, as it was when he had Guillain–Barré syndrome 10 years ago.

ON EXAMINATION

- Coarse skin
- Rattling chest
- Beefy, red tongue
- Downgoing left plantar; right plantar is equivocal
- Guttering between the metacarpals of both hands
- Wax blocking left ear
- Right pupil = 3 mm diameter; left pupil = 4 mm diameter. Both react well to light.
- Forehead furrowed
- Eyebrows raised

a) **What is the diagnosis?**

OK. This is easy enough for some. As always, there is much evidence given to try to confuse. The paint story is to make you think about toxic solvents. The past Guillain–Barré syndrome is a red herring. The inclusion of dry skin is probably an effort to make you think of myxoedema. Wax in the ear – ignore it. Here the trick is to tease out what we really know to be the abnormalities, and they have been deliberately obscured. We know that a hand is weak, and that there is 'guttering'. This tells us that he has wasting of the intrinsic muscles of the hands, which are supplied by T1. Could this be a T1 lesion in a smoker? Yes. This is a classic case of Pancoast tumour. What about the eye? One pupil is definitely smaller than the other. The eyebrows are raised, which suggests compensation for a ptosis. Ptosis plus a small pupil suggests a classic Horner's syndrome.

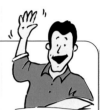

A4   **a) Diagnosis**
So, we have a slight variation. You have had to spot two classic cases and put them together. The patient has a Pancoast tumour with ipsilateral Horner's syndrome – a classic case in itself.

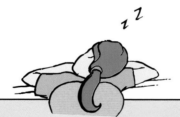

REVISION ZONE

These classics rely upon a knowledge of the typical pupillary syndromes, of which there are four: Horner's syndrome, third nerve palsy, Argyll Robertson pupil, and Holmes–Adie syndrome. So let's have a look at these.

Horner's corner, tramps, ladies of the night, and hermits

(Little Jack) Horner's syndrome

How would you feel if you had just stuck in your thumb and pulled out a plum? Just like Miss Muffitt sitting on her tuffet, this might generate some form of sympathetic response. Facially, you might be expected to go wide-eyed, sweaty, and for your eyes to pop out like organ stops. Loss of sympathetic activity (causing Horner's syndrome) produces the exact opposite – a sunken eye (enophthalmos) with a small pupil, partial ptosis, and ipsilateral loss of sweating. The course of the sympathetic supply may be interrupted at one of two main points:

- its origin: stroke, syrinx, tumour, encephalitis, multiple sclerosis (MS) plaque, or anything else in the surgical sieve that might hit the brainstem
- the neck: carotid aneurysm, Pancoast tumour, or trauma

Alternatively, the features and causes can be remembered another way:

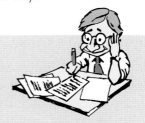

Little Jack Horner, 'e SSAT* in the Corner
There with his sunken eye
His small pupil hid
'neath his poor drooping lid
with the side of his face crisp and dry!'

*Encephalitis, Stroke, Syrinx, Aneurysm of the carotid, Tumour (including Pancoast), Trauma

A congenital Horner's syndrome is benign and often associated with heterochromia (one iris differs in colour from the other).

Tramps

Why is a third nerve palsy known as the tramps' palsy? Because of the complete ptosis or the dilated pupil? No; it is because the eye is found to be looking 'down and out'!

Third nerve palsy complicates the diagnosis of raised intracranial pressure, as the third nerve stretches under the uncus and palsy produces a false lateralising sign. Equally, in the presence of a headache (painful third nerve palsy) the diagnosis is of a rapidly expanding posterior communicating artery aneurysm until proven otherwise; this is a reason for immediate admission and computed tomography (CT) scan or magnetic resonance imaging (MRI). The pupil is frequently involved, as the parasympathetic fibres from the Edinger–Westphal nucleus to the pupil lie on the outside of the third nerve where they are vulnerable to an expanding mass. Diabetes mellitus can cause a palsy that is usually painless. Diabetes can cause inflammation or thrombosis of the vasa nervorum to the third nerve, which predominantly affects the central nerve fibres of the third nerve, hence resulting in pupillary sparing.

Examinations often refer to Weber's syndrome (third nerve palsy with contralateral hemiplegia), which is due to a basilar artery event causing infarction of a cerebral peduncle.

Put another way, **the causes** *of a third nerve palsy* are those that damage the origin of the nerve in the midbrain (e.g. midbrain amyloid, MS, Weber's syndrome), and those that damage the nerve vasculature (e.g. diabetes, vasculitis due to systemic lupus erythematosus [SLE], rheumatoid arthritis [RA], polyarteritis nodosa), and nerve compression and stretch (e.g. posterior cerebral artery aneurysms, tumours). Transient and repetitive paroxysmal third nerve palsies can occur with migraines.

Ladies of the night

The Argyll Robertson pupil was classically said to be due to syphilis and, in a weak pun, earned the name of the prostitute's pupil, as it does not like the light much, but is very accommodating; it is characterised by small irregular pupils that do not react to light, but do accommodate. This is a little unfair, now that the commonest cause is diabetes mellitus. Other aetiologies include: long-standing Adie's syndrome, encephalitis, amyloidosis, mid-brain tumours (e.g. pinealoma), sarcoidosis, Lyme disease, and the presence of chronic iritis.

Hermits

Holmes–Adie pupil usually occurs in women, and is mostly unilateral. It is characterised by a myotonic pupil – a dilated pupil that responds sluggishly to light. Unlike the Argyll Robertson pupil, the hermit's Holmes–Adie pupil does not like the light much (if at all), and is not very accommodating, although it can be persuaded to accommodate slowly. Knee and ankle jerks may be absent.

CAUSES OF A DILATED PUPIL (MYDRIASIS)

- Topical mydriatic drugs (e.g. atropine, homatropine, tropicamide, cyclopentolate)
- Sympathomimetic drugs (e.g. amphetamines)
- Anticholinergic drugs (e.g. tricyclic antidepressants)
- Third nerve lesion (note some lesions may be pupillary sparing)
- Holmes–Adie syndrome
- Phaeochromocytoma
- Retrobulbar neuritis/optic atrophy
- Iridectomy
- Congenital

CAUSES OF A CONSTRICTED PUPIL (MIOSIS)

- Drugs: opiates (reversed by naloxone), parasympathomimetics (e.g. pilocarpine), organophosphate toxicity, cholinesterase inhibitors, phenothiazines
- Pontine haemorrhage (obtunded patient with Cheyne–Stokes respiration and focal neurological signs)
- Encephalitis
- Horner's syndrome
- Iritis and keratitis
- Argyll Robertson pupil
- Sleep and sedatives
- Congenital

Q5 You are asked to examine a 23-year-old woman with recurrent headaches on one of the medical wards. She has had the headaches for about 1 year, and they have occurred at all times of the day. She denies any paraesthesia, but has complained of an occasional episode of blurred vision. No episodes of loss of consciousness have occurred. According to her medical history, she had mild asthma as a child, suffered from a prolonged attack of measles at the age of four years, and suffered whiplash in a road traffic accident 5 years ago. Her father and paternal grandfather suffered from migraine. Her only medication at the moment is the oral contraceptive pill, which she has been taking for 7 years. Apart from the occasional muscle ache after exercise, she admits to no other symptoms. She has two jobs – one working in a cake shop by day and one on a petrol forecourt in the evenings – which she finds very stressful.

On examination she is 5 ft tall and weighs 120 kg. Her blood pressure is 132/72 mmHg and she has a pulse of 91 beats/minute. The results of examination of the respiratory and cardiovascular systems are unremarkable. Her reflexes are normal and her plantar response is downgoing. Apart from some slight difficulty with past-pointing, she has no other cerebellar signs. Fundoscopy shows that both disc margins are blurred, but she has no signs of other retinopathy. Her gastrointestinal examination is normal.

Investigations	Results
Urea and electrolytes	Normal
Full blood count	Normal
Serum calcium/phosphate	Normal
Arterial blood gas analysis	Normal
Chest X-ray	Normal
CT scan of head	Unremarkable
MRI	Normal
Lumbar puncture	No oligoclonal bands

a) What is the most likely diagnosis?

b) What are the three most important steps in her management?

There are a myriad of red herrings here – stress, past head injury, and a family history of migraine, to name but a few. There is *only* one finding that is always pathological, and for which there is a limited list of causes, and this is papilloedema. Write down your list now.

Don't look down – no cheating!

Once you have established that she is not hypertensive and has no respiratory problems and excluded the possibility of mass lesions and multiple sclerosis through investigations, then the diagnosis should be easy. *She is of entirely normal weight* – for someone 7 ft tall! To anyone else, she is at best 'vertically and nutritionally challenged'. In addition, she takes the oral contraceptive pill. Together, these facts should swing you towards a diagnosis of benign intracranial hypertension. The only problem left to you now is to know the management. Being the MRCP examination, it is tempting to think of the most bizarre forms of treatment. In reality, the examiners would like you to be sensible. Do not be too clever.

A: Papilloedema

- benign intracranial pressure
- malignant hypertension
- mass lesions
- hypercapnia
- central retinal vein or cavernous sinus thrombosis
- hydrocephalus
- vitamin A toxicity
- lead poisoning and optic neuritis

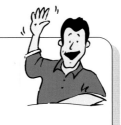

A5 a) **Diagnosis**
Benign intracranial hypertension
(multiple sclerosis = no marks)

b) **Management**
Lose weight
- Stop the oral contraceptive pill
- Start acetazolamide (or loop/thiazide diuretics)

You may also
- Start prednisolone
- Repeat lumbar punctures with removal of cerebrospinal fluid (CSF)

FOR THE RECORD

Benign intracranial hypertension is also known as pseudotumour cerebri. It occurs most frequently in women aged 15–44 years. There are many presumptive risk factors, most notably a high body mass index (obesity), pregnancy, and the oral contraceptive pill. Other associations used in MRCP examinations include the use of tetracyclines (e.g. patients treated for acne), corticosteroids, or lithium.

Q6 A 23-year-old woman presents to her GP with headache, nausea, and vomiting. She works as a cleaner in a local supermarket. She is married with three children. She had an appendectomy at the age of 6 years and has complained of dysmenorrhoea since her periods started at the age of 14 years. She is otherwise relatively fit and well. Examination reveals bilateral blurring of the optic discs. She has a mild degree of past-pointing bilaterally on testing, and a broad-based gait. Otherwise examination of the nervous system is unremarkable. Her blood pressure is 120/90 mm Hg; she has a pulse rate of 90 beats/minute. Clinical examination including gynaecological examination is otherwise entirely normal.

INVESTIGATIONS	RESULTS
Plasma sodium	132 mmol/l
Plasma potassium	3.9 mmol/l
Plasma bicarbonate	24 mmol/l
Plasma urea	4.3 mmol/l
Plasma glucose	3.6 mmol/l
Haemoglobin	20.2 g/dl
White cell count	3.6×10^9/l
Platelets	189×10^9/l
ESR	1 mm in first hour
Kidneys	Normal
Liver	Normal
Spleen	Normal
Ovaries and uterus	Appear normal

a) What three tests would you do next?

b) Why is the ESR only 1?

c) What is the most likely diagnosis?

Cover the page below, and read line by line.

Here we go again!

First, what are the key findings that are *always* abnormal and for which there are a defined list of causes? Write them down.

Now, which diagnosis appears on all lists?

Don't turn over until you have finished your lists, and come up with your answer.

Your list here…

This question requires you to notice that this patient has a grossly abnormal elevated haemoglobin level and papilloedema.

Papilloedema

Papilloedema may be benign (benign intracranial pressure, which of course isn't benign) or malignant (malignant hypertension or tumour). Other causes include:

- mass lesions in (abscess or benign tumour) or around (e.g. chronic subdural) the brain
- too much blood getting in: hypercapnia causes loss of cerebral autoregulation
- too little blood getting out: central retinal vein, sagittal sinus, or cavernous sinus thrombosis
- too little CSF getting out: hydrocephalus including post-subarachnoid haemorrhage
- lead poisoning and optic neuritis

Polycythaemia

Relative
- dehydration
- Gaisböck's syndrome (stress)

Primary
- polycythaemia rubra vera (splenomegaly, raised platelets)

Secondary
- hypoxia
- chronic obstructive pulmonary disease
- altitude
- abnormal haemoglobins
- sleep apnoea

Excess erythropoietin
- cerebellar haemangioma
- hepatoma
- phaeochromocytoma
- hypernephroma
- polycystic/transplant kidneys
- uterine leiomyoma/fibroma

Working it out

This is a tricky question, and takes our thoughts to a slightly higher and 'more devious' level. Clearly, any 'true' polycythaemia causes hyperviscosity and can lead to cerebral vessel thrombosis, whether cavernous sinus, sagittal sinus, or central vein. These can all cause papilloedema, and so all causes of true polycythaemia suddenly become candidates. However, the membership examination is usually not *quite* so stupid: if there were this many right answers, then the paper would be impossible to mark. There is usually a 'list overlap', or a clue, and in this case, both are present.

Something is going on in the cerebellum (the clues being the past-pointing and balance). You will know all the signs of cerebellar disease – they were first comprehensively described by Gordon Holmes (Professor of Neurology at the National Hospital for Neurology, Queen Square, UK) based on his meticulous observations of soldiers with cerebellar bullet wounds in the First World War. These signs include atonia (low tone), ataxia, overshoot, asynergy and dysdiadochokinesis, past-pointing and intention tremor, along with broad-based gait, impaired eye movements including nystagmus (towards the lesion), and scanning speech. Remember that these signs are predominantly from the cerebellar hemispheres, not the vermis. Midline (or vermis) lesions often have none of these signs, but such patients are troubled by truncal ataxia or the inability to maintain posture, along with marked nausea, vomiting, and vertigo.

> *"Blokes who have strokes at the back of the brain*
> *Will vomit and say they can't walk straight again*
> *Ataxic: nystagmic: past-point finger-nose*
> *Intent on a tremor, they scan with their prose*
> *If hit in the vermis they all comb their hair*
> *Instead they can't walk or sit down on a chair."*

So, are there any cerebellar problems on the 'polycythaemic' list? Yes! Cerebellar haemangioblastomas are seen in von Hippel–Lindau syndrome.

Does this fit with the list of causes of papilloedema? Yes – a vascular tumour. Of course, you could have reached the same conclusion by using your list of causes of cerebellar syndromes. Write one down now. We shall be telling you what the list is in a moment.

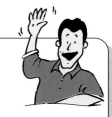

A6

a) **Investigations**
CT or MRI scan of the brain
Total red cell volume/red cell mass
Bone marrow biopsy with trephine
Urine/blood erythropoietin level

b) **ESR = 1**
ESR is low in the presence of polycythaemia

c) **Diagnosis**
Cerebellar haemangioblastoma (von Hippel–Lindau syndrome)

QUIZ SPOT!

Q: What are the causes of very low ESR?

A: Polycythaemia
Afibrinogenaemia and hypofibrinogenaemia
Remember, as a simple rule the ESR should be age ÷ 2 (and in females, add 10 to the result).

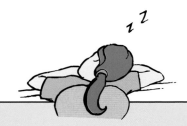

REVISION ZONE
The eyes have it!
We have had a nice (common) case of papilloedema. You now need to remind yourself of the other common problems at the back of the eye.

OPTIC ATROPHY (THE PALLID DISC)
Write down your list of causes in the space below. Then check it against ours (which follows).

Your list here...

OUR LIST

In the **p**resence of **p**allor **p**osterior to the **p**upil, **p**roceed to **p**eruse **p**aediatrics (Friedreich's ataxia, Leber's optic atrophy, and Wolfram's syndrome [DIDMOAD – diabetes insipidus, diabetes mellitus, optic atrophy, and deafness] are the main congenital ones to remember), **p**apilloedema (longstanding), **p**ressure (e.g. compression by tumour and glaucoma), **p**oisons (quinine overdose, tobacco amblyopia, wood alcohol), **P**aget's disease, **p**ernicious anaemia and **p**oor diet (vitamin B_{12} deficiency), **p**ulselessness (retinal artery ischaemia), **p**syphilis, and **p**multiple sclerosis (it is a little known fact that these last two have a silent 'p').

Now list the causes of papilloedema (already learnt; see page 29)...

_____

_____

_____

_____

_____

_____

_____

_____

_____

_____

_____

_____

_____

_____

_____

_____

Angioid retinal streaks

These are seen as visible thickening and calcification of the elastic layer of Bruch's membrane. The causes may be remembered as the female who is doing a streak.

"... *perhaps* she *shall* bi*cycle acro*ss the road with *her elastic* loose"

or

"...*Paget's* she *thal* bi*sickle acro* the road with *Ehlers elasticum* loose"

Paget's disease, thalassaemia, sickle cell anaemia, acromegaly, Ehlers–Danlos syndrome, pseudoxanthoma elasticum

Pseudoxanthoma elasticum

- recessive or dominant inheritance of a defect in a cholesterol transporter gene
- the recipe for 'chicken skin' lesions? Saggy skin with buttery papules and plaques (seen in the face, neck, axilla, antecubital fossa, popliteal fossa, and groin)
- cardiovascular complications include premature vascular disease with claudication or myocardial infarction

CHOROIDORETINITIS

Repeat after me:

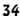

Choroid makes it hard to see
when hit with all the nasty three:
but sarcoid, syphilis, TB
with tox may go, and CMV!

CMV: cytomegalovirus; sarcoid: sarcoidosis; TB: tuberculosis; tox: toxoplasmosis and toxocariasis

Retinitis pigmentosa

Remember that retinitis pigmentosa usually affects the peripheral retina, sparing the macula and, therefore, resulting in tunnel vision.

Diseases associated with retinitis pigmentosa (corpuscular retinal pigmentation) are:

- hereditary ataxias such as Friedreich's ataxia, an autosomal recessive or sex-linked condition. Spinal cord atrophy occurs with degeneration of the spinocerebellar tracts (hence cerebellar signs), corticospinal tracts (hence long-tract signs), and dorsal columns. Peripheral neuropathies make this one of the causes of extensor plantars and absent ankle jerks. It also causes a cardiomyopathy, scoliosis and pes cavus
- Refsum's disease: an autosomal recessive neuropathy causing anosmia, deafness, and sensory neuropathy, with cerebellar ataxia and a high CSF protein concentration
- Laurence–Moon–Biedl syndrome: an autosomal recessive disorder characterised by obesity, polydactyly, intellectual retardation, hypogonadism and renal dysgenesis, diabetes mellitus, and endocrinopathies
- Alport's syndrome: hereditary nephritis
- Kearns–Sayre syndrome: a mitochondrial disease caused by deletions of mitochondrial DNA – note the link with mitochondria
- Usher's syndrome: causes sensorineural hearing impairment
- abetalipoproteinaemia and vitamin E deficiency

A QUICK JOKE

A woman accompanied her husband to the doctor, on account of his failing vision. Afterwards, the doctor takes the wife aside. "Do all I say, or your husband will go blind. You must make him his favourite breakfast each morning, to set him up for the day. In the evening, let him relax while you prepare a sumptuous five-course spread. Don't let him do any household chores. Have sex with him as often as he likes, and fulfil his every whim and fancy – no matter how depraved!"

On the way home, the husband turns to his wife. "I saw the doctor take you aside. Is everything going to be OK?"

"No," she replied, "you're going to go blind."

Before we move on...

Have a quick think. Can you remember:

- the causes of polyarthralgia?

_____

_____

_____

_____

- the revised Duckett–Jones criteria?

_____

_____

_____

_____

- all about the three phases of Lyme disease?

_____

_____

_____

_____

Can you write down the surgical sieve?

_____

_____

_____

_____

_____

_____

Now check your answers against the lists: causes of polyarthralgia (page 5), the revised Duckett—Jones criteria (page 7), the three phases of Lyme disease (page 10), and the surgical sieve (pages 13–14)

BRAIN BITS AND CORD CHUNKS

Cerebellar syndromes

Remind yourself of the clinical features. In particular, is the nystagmus oscillation towards or away from the lesion? Remember that vermis lesions are different. Can you recite the verse you should have learnt (page 30)?

For the causes of cerebellar syndromes, go through the usual surgical sieve, but remember: they need a: **FAT CAT S**can for **MS.**

Friedreich's ataxia:
Alcohol*
Tumours: primary: cerebellar haemangioblastomas
                                von Hippel–Lindau syndrome
        secondary: especially lung cancer as a paraneoplastic syndrome
Congenital: **a**taxia **t**elangiectasia and Arnold–Chiari malformations
Strokes
MS

Rarer causes of cerebellar syndromes include:

- metabolic causes (thiamine deficiency, hypothyroidism)
- drugs and toxins (phenytoin, barbiturates, alcoholism, lead poisoning)

Note that ataxia telangiectasia is associated with immunodeficiency, cancer susceptibility, radiosensitivity, and elevated serum alphafetoprotein levels.

---

* Alcohol abuse causes cerebellar degeneration. Strangely, this happens to us acutely and reversibly, with 10 pints of finest lager causing ataxia, slurred speech, nausea and vertigo. This syndrome – known to experts as 'bed spin' – is poorly detailed in standard texts. You can try it out for yourselves on the night that you pass this damned examination. You'll find that we are right.

SPASTIC PARAPARESIS

Anatomically, there are few options for the site of the lesion. Being spastic, it has to be an upper motor neurone problem. The only site that will hit both legs (only) is across the spinal cord, or parasagitally with something (usually a parasagittal meningioma) pressing on the cortical motor strip. If there are no sensory signs at all, then the latter is the most likely diagnosis, especially if there are any other signs above the foramen magnum (such as raised intracranial pressure, epilepsy, or other focal neurology). If there is a sensory level deficit and no signs above the foramen magnum, a cord lesion is more likely. Use your sieve to produce a list of cord lesion causes:

OK? FINISHED?

Well, barring all the usual causes of cord compression, the main ones (and those which people miss) are:

- transverse myelitis complicating a viral infection (such as HIV), MS, or a paraneoplastic syndrome
- sudden vascular occlusion: this can be due to compression by a tumour or extradural abscess, or secondary to a vasculitis. In the case of an abscess or tumour, there may not be loss of a complete sensory level (e.g. posterior columns may be spared).
- tropical spastic paraparesis: this is a complication of human T-cell lymphoma virus (HTLV) I/III infection, the other complication of which is lymphoma. It is most commonly seen in those of Afro–Caribbean descent, and presents with a very slow (over decades) paralysis after initial backache and constipation

ABSENT ANKLE JERKS, EXTENSOR PLANTARS

Work out your own way of remembering this list of causes. As to whether it is actually any use is debatable; nobody we know ever remembers this turning up as a part II question. The main causes are:

- syringomyelia
- taboparesis (syphilis)
- Friedreich's ataxia
- cervical spondylosis and peripheral neuropathy
- motor neurone disease
- subacute combined degeneration of the cord

BRAIN JUICE

Look out for the following changes:

Lymphocytosis

Think 'inflammation without ordinary bacteria'. Work your way through your surgical sieve, and write a list, then compare it with ours.

Your list here...

_____

_____

_____

_____

_____

_____

_____

_____

_____

_____

_____

_____

_____

_____

_____

_____

OUR LIST

The 'not ordinary bacteria' list includes all the 'odd-ball' infections:

* Viruses (including HIV)
* Fungi
* Syphilis
* *Rickettsia* (Lyme disease, caused by *Borrelia burgdorferi*)
* *Listeria*
* *Brucella*
* *Coxiella*
* *Mycoplasma*
* Whipple's disease

Abscess and tuberculous meningitis/encephalitis are the ones most commonly found in the MRCP examination.

The 'not infections at all' list includes:

* Tumours
* MS
* SLE
* Sarcoidosis
* Behçet's syndrome

Remember, there are some catches. Cerebral lymphoproliferative disease can produce CSF full of 'lymphocytes'. A woman treated with steroids for more than 1 year for flares of cerebral sarcoidosis (MRI had suggested cerebral sarcoidosis, and the CSF was full of lymphocytes) complained of gum bleeding when brushing her teeth. A blood film showed her to have acute lymphoblastic leukaemia (ALL). The cells in the CSF were not lymphocytes, but mature lymphoblasts. She had responded well to steroids, which are very good at killing lymphoblasts.

Another catch? A partially treated bacterial meningitis may present with a CSF lymphocytosis.

RAISED PROTEIN, NORMAL CSF CELLS

Note that Guillain–Barré syndrome is a motor neuropathy occurring after an infection (often viral). It can be recurrent. The catches? Well, they can sell it to you as respiratory failure, and with sensory symptoms (although *signs* are usually absent). Beware, also, that the presence of a raised CSF cell count (especially lymphocytosis) is *not* compatible with Guillan–Barré syndrome, although a raised CSF protein is compatible. The other causes of a raised CSF protein with normal cell count are lead poisoning, cord compression, spinal block (Froin's syndrome), cord malignant deposits, syphilis, and subacute sclerosing panencephalitis.

Is Part II getting on your nerves yet?

Peripheral polyneuropathy

Here is one way of remembering the list.

Born unlucky:	Friedreich's ataxia, Refsum's disease, Charcot–Marie–Tooth disease

Three dejected:
- alcoholics due to the effects of alcohol
- vitamin B_1, B_6, and B_{12} deficiencies
- isoniazid used to treat TB – which is why people receiving TB treatment must receive pyridoxine supplements

Two infected:
- leprosy
- Guillain–Barré syndrome*

Two injected:
- paraneoplasia* in cancer patients, or the effects of its treatments, such as vincristine and isoniazid
- diabetes mellitus

One connected:	connective tissue disease, such as RA/SLE/polyarteritis nodosa
Granuloma suspected:	sarcoidosis, Churg–Strauss syndrome, and (hypothyroid which just refuses to rhyme).

Sometimes, there is a motor neuropathy alone. This may be due to the **d**uo starred* causes above (**d**iabetic amyotrophy and **d**iphtheria), **p**orphyria (acute intermittent), **p**olymyositis, or **l**ead poisoning.

Another way of classifying neuropathies is as follows:

AXONAL	DEMYELINATING	MONONEURITIS MULTIPLEX
• HSMN type I	• HSMN type II	• Diabetes mellitus
• Diabetes mellitus	• Diabetes mellitus	• Leprosy
• B_{12} deficiency	• B_{12} deficiency	• Connective tissue diseases:
• Folate deficiency	• Paraprotein neuropathy	e.g. PAN, SLE, RA, GCA
• Renal failure	• Inflammation:	• Sarcoidosis
• Carcinomatous neuropathy	Guillain–Barré syndrome	• Malignancy
• Porphyria	and chronic inflammatory	• Amyloidosis
• Amyloidosis	demyelinating neuropathy	• Neurofibromatosis
• Toxins (e.g. phenytoin,		• HIV/AIDS
isoniazid, nitrofurantoin,		• Churg–Strauss syndrome
dapsone, organophosphate,		
vincristine, alcohol, heavy		
metals)		
• HIV		
• Critical care neuropathy		

GCA: giant cell arteritis; HSMN: hereditary sensory and motor neuropathy; PAN: polyarteritis nodosa; RA: rheumatoid arthritis; SLE: systemic lupus erythematosus

You can make up your own ways of remembering these, if you want!

CARPAL TUNNEL SYNDROME

The causes 'have got to be PRAM' (have gout **TB P²RA³M**).

Gout, **TB**, **p**regnancy/**p**ill, **r**heumatoid **a**rthritis and **a**cromegaly/**a**myloidosis, and **m**yxoedema. Renal disease is said to be another '**r**', and diabetes mellitus may be associated through amyloidosis.

Quiz Spot!

Q: Abdominal pain and peripheral neuropathy ought to flag up two classic membership thoughts. What are they?

A: Lead poisoning and acute intermittent porphyria

Phew! Time for a drink and a break

When you start again, make sure that you have all of these lists completely sorted before you move on. This should be your habit on working through the book. Whenever you start again, run through **all** the lists you have learnt up to that point, and make sure that you still have them off pat.

But before we finish, another quick joke...

As the businessman aged, he suffered increasingly frequent and severe headaches. He sought specialist help. The neurologist examined him thoroughly. "You have a one-in-a-million condition in which your testicles are pressed against the base of your spine. I can cure your headaches," he said, "but this will require castration. The way to relieve the pressure – and hence the headache – is to remove the testicles." Recognising the seriousness of the condition, the businessman felt that he had no choice.

With a clear mind (no headache and a considerably lighter undercarriage) the man left hospital after the operation. To cheer himself up, he decided to buy a suit. The salesman looked at him and, without blinking, said "Size 42 long." "Correct! How did you know?" The suit fitted perfectly. "It's my job. New shirt?" said the salesman, "34 sleeve and $15^1/_2$ collar?" "Yes, and correct!" said the man, "how did you know?" "It's my job. Shoes? Size 10?" "Yes! Amazing! Perfect fit! How did you know?" "It's my job". "How about new underwear? Size 36?" "No" said the man. "I always wear size 34!" "Oh, no! no! no!" he said. "You can't do that! It will push your testicles against the base of your spine and give you a hell of a headache."

NEUROLOGY CLASSICS

Finally, there are some 'classic cases' that you ought to recognise. Here they are!

Friedreich's ataxia

This is characterised by absent ankle jerks/extensor plantars, cerebellar ataxia, pyramidal tract disease, dorsal column/spinocerebellar sensory neuropathy, pes cavus, and optic atrophy.

It is associated with hypertrophic cardiomyopathy in up to 90% of patients, diabetes mellitus in 10%–20%, and various other features including: sensorineural deafness, marfanoid features (kyphoscoliosis and high-arched palate), low IQ, and retinitis pigmentosa. Patients usually present early in their teens with debilitating neurology and die in their fourth decade of cardiac failure. They may appear as a case of 'absent ankle jerks and upgoing plantars' or dementia.

Guillain–Barré syndrome

This is characterised by viral/coryzal illness, demyelinating neuropathy (sensory or motor), and bulbar weakness. The Miller–Fisher variant of the Guillain–Barré syndrome is characterised by viral/coryzal illness, external ophthalmoplegia, descending motor neuropathy, and sensory ataxia

Both Guillain–Barré syndrome and Miller–Fisher syndrome have a very high CSF protein. Other causes of a demyelinating neuropathy include: diabetes mellitus, vitamin B_{12} deficiency, diphtheria, and Charcot–Marie–Tooth disease.

Hartnup disease

This is characterised by convulsions, cerebellar signs, mental retardation, diarrhoea, and photosensitivity.

Huntington's disease

This is characterised by chorea, akinesia, rigidity, dementia, and genetic anticipation.

Laurence–Moon–Biedl syndrome

This is characterised by retinitis pigmentosa, mental retardation, obesity, hypogonadism, and polydactyly. It is also associated with dwarfism and renal defects.

Refsum's disease

This is characterised by sensorimotor neuropathy, cerebellar ataxia, retinitis pigmentosa, and deafness. It is also associated with cataracts and ichthyosis (scaly skin). Like Friedreich's ataxia, it is also associated with cardiomyopathy and optic atrophy. Unlike Friedreich's ataxia, however, the symptoms of Refsum's are reversible with a low phytanic acid diet.

Shy–Drager syndrome

This is characterised by parkinsonism (tremor, rigidity, and bradykinesia), and primary autonomic failure (e.g. postural hypotension).

NB: This is now part of the multi-system atrophy syndrome (MSA).

Steele–Richardson–Olszewski syndrome

This is characterised by parkinsonism (with marked axial rigidity), progressive supranuclear palsy, frontal lobe features, and dementia.

Wilson's disease

This is characterised by parkinsonism/dementia in younger patients, jaundice/cirrhosis, and proximal renal tubular acidosis

Note that it is an autosomal recessive disease that causes failure of copper secretion into bile, hence causing acute liver failure, chronic hepatitis, or cirrhosis. The diagnosis is based upon decreased serum caeruloplasmin, increased urinary copper, haemolytic anaemia, slit lamp investigations that reveal Kayser–Fleischer rings, and liver biopsy. Treatment is copper chelation with penicillamine.

Sturge–Weber syndrome

This is characterised by port-wine stain, epilepsy, optic atrophy, choroid angioma, and squint.

Wallenberg's syndrome

This is characterised by ipsilateral Horner's syndrome/cerebellar signs/dysphagia/dysarthria/ trigeminal pain, contralateral spinothalamic sensory loss/mild hemiparesis, and hiccough. It is also known as lateral medullary syndrome or posterior inferior cerebellar artery syndrome. It usually presents with acute vertigo and vomiting.

Wernicke's encephalopathy

This is characterised by cerebellar ataxia, ophthalmoplegia with nystagmus, peripheral sensory neuropathy, and, of course, heavy alcohol use. It is largely due to thiamine/vitamin B₁ deficiency. A confirmatory test is an assay of red cell transketolase, which is reduced when thiamine is deficient. Some laboratories can now perform direct red cell thiamine assays.

Acute intermittent porphyria

This is characterised by peripheral motor neuropathy, papilloedema, abdominal pain, and syndrome of inappropriate secretion of ADH (SIADH). It is also associated with epilepsy in 20% of patients, fever, sinus tachycardia, hypertension, hypercholesterolaemia, psychosis, and, not surprisingly, depression!

Chronic lead poisoning

This is characterised by peripheral motor neuropathy, papilloedema/optic atrophy, abdominal pain, convulsions, aseptic meningitis, sideroblastic anaemia, chronic interstitial nephritis, and a blue line on the gums.

Note that high lead levels result in raised porphyrin levels due to an interruption of porphyrin metabolism. So, if the information given does not seem to fit with any of the porphyrias, think lead! Don't forget that lead poisoning also produces basophilic stippling on the blood film. In the MRCP examination, it occurs in plumbers, painters, or children with a pica for paint! It is treated with intravenous penicillamine, which acts as a chelating agent.

Langerhans cell histiocytosis (histiocytosis X)

This is characterised by cranial diabetes insipidus, otitis externa, exophthalmos, rash, and lytic lesions on skull X-ray.

Tuberous sclerosis

This is characterised by epilepsy, mental retardation, adenoma sebaceum, subungual fibromata, café-au-lait spots, ash-leaf macules, and shagreen patches. It is associated with a higher than normal incidence of malignancy, in particular, retinal phakomas, renal and pulmonary hamartomas, and rhabdomyosarcomas.

Syringomyelia

This is characterised by lower limb spastic paraparesis, upper limb lower motor neurone weakness/wasting, Horner's syndrome, nystagmus, and 'balaclava' sensory loss.

Note that sneezing and coughing both increase intracerebral pressure and therefore result in exacerbation of symptoms in syringomyelia. It can also be associated with neural tube defects (e.g. myelomeningocele), a tethered spinal cord, and a Chiari malformation of the skull and brainstem.

Phenylketonuria (PKU)

This is characterised by epilepsy, mental retardation, and hypopigmentation. PKU is routinely screened for in the UK on day 5 following birth using the Guthrie test. If positive, the treatment is a low alanine diet in the first few months of life.

von Hippel–Lindau syndrome

This is characterised by retinal angiomas, cerebellar signs due to cerebellar haemangioblastomas, and polycythaemia due to excess erythropoietin production. It is an autosomal dominant disease.

Mollaret's meningitis

This is characterised by recurrent episodes of aseptic meningitis associated with recurrent herpetic infection, raised CSF pressure, and CSF lymphocytosis.

3

PANTS

RESPIRATORY MRCP LISTS

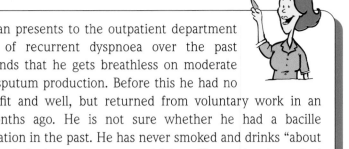

Q7 A 63-year-old man presents to the outpatient department with a history of recurrent dyspnoea over the past 6 months. He finds that he gets breathless on moderate exertion, but has not had any sputum production. Before this he had no respiratory illnesses and was fit and well, but returned from voluntary work in an orphanage in Tasmania 8 months ago. He is not sure whether he had a bacille Calmette–Guérin (BCG) vaccination in the past. He has never smoked and drinks "about 8 pints on a Saturday". He is married with two grown-up children. He previously worked in the aerospace industry and had a brief spell of no more than 2 years in the atomic industry. Before he retired he had also worked in a local newsagents shop. He denies any asbestos contact, fevers, weight loss, haemoptysis, skin rashes, or arthralgia. He has no history of epilepsy. He has never had any renal tract problems, although he admits to symptoms of prostatism. On examination, he appears well and has no evidence of lymphadenopathy. He has a blood pressure of 130/80 mm Hg and a pulse of 72 beats/min. He has no neurological signs and the abdominal examination is unremarkable. Fine crepitations can be heard at both lung bases.

Investigations

Investigations	Results
FBC	Normal
Liver function tests	Aspartate aminotransferase 32 IU/l (5–15)
	Alanine aminotransferase 23 IU/l (5–15)
	Bilirubin 6 μmol/l
	Alkaline phosphatase 95 IU/l
Serum calcium	2.32 mmol/l
Serum ACE	Normal
Echocardiography	Good LV function, valves appear normal
Chest: X-ray	Bilateral hilar lymphadenopathy, with midzone reticulonodular shadowing. No evidence of cavitation
Lung function tests	K_{CO} 72%
	FEV_1 1.8 l
	FVC 2.1 l
	DLCO 70% predicted
Urinalysis and electrolytes	Normal
Abdominal ultrasound	Normal
Liver biopsy	No evidence of malignancy, possible granuloma seen

ACE: angiotensin converting enzyme; DLCO: carbon monoxide diffusion in the lung; FEV_1: forced expiratory volume in 1 second; FBC: full blood count; FVC: forced vital capacity; KCO: transfer co-efficient of carbon monoxide. Figures in parentheses indicate normal ranges.

a) What are the two most likely diagnoses?

b) What two investigations would you use to confirm the diagnosis?

Although there is a lot of information in this question, the two most obvious problems are the presence of bilateral hilar lymphadenopathy (BHL) and restrictive lung function with other features of fibrosis. If we revise the causes of these two problems then the diagnosis should become apparent.

First of all – as usual – jot down the lists of causes as best you can in the space below:

Your list here...

BHL	Restrictive lung function

Causes of BHL

You will have to make up your own way of remembering this list. Fortunately, it is short: 'Two pairs are CCHEAPP': there are two pairs of obvious causes and six less obvious causes. Obvious causes (two pairs) include sarcoidosis and tuberculosis (TB), and lymphoma and cancers. The six less obvious causes (CCHEAPP) are cystic fibrosis/Churg–Strauss syndrome, HIV, extrinsic alveolitis, phenytoin treatment, and pneumoconiosis (especially berylliosis). Remember that Churg–Strauss syndrome may have glomerulonephritis, gut involvement causing ulcers and diarrhoea, skin involvement, and mononeuritis multiplex.

Causes of lung fibrosis

Any chronic diffuse lung inflammation will, in general, cause fibrosis. Any toxic agent may produce damage directly. Otherwise, the main causes are shown below.

Main causes of lung fibrosis:

- TB
- drugs: amiodarone, bleomycin, busulphan, etc.
- pneumoconioses: silicosis, asbestosis
- acute rheumatic disease (RA, SLE, etc.)
- radiation
- sarcoidosis
- hypersensitivity pneumonitis (pigeon breeders lung, etc.)
- paraquat
- pulmonary haemosiderosis
- histiocytosis X

Remember: Pigeon CRA³PS: cryptogenic fibrosing alveolitis (CFA)*, radiation, amiodarone, (extrinsic) allergic alveolitis, pigeon breeders lung, sarcoidosis

*Remember that CFA is associated with other autoimmune diseases, especially rheumatoid arthritis (RA), ankylosing spondylitis, Sjögren's syndrome, chronic active hepatitis (CAH), Hashimoto's disease, and inflammatory bowel disease, and also with renal tubular acidosis. In essence, this is the same list as that for the associations of chronic active hepatitis (see later, under 'gastroenterological lists'), so learn it only once! It is associated with clubbing, and (like CAH) positive antinuclear antibodies and antimitochondrial antibodies.

Also sneaking in there as other causes of a cellular lung infiltrate and fibrosis are the histiocytosis X files:

- eosinophilic granuloma
- Hand–Schüller–Christian disease
- Letterer–Siwe disease: hepatosplenomegaly, anaemia, diabetes insipidus, Rhesus factor positive, pulmonary hypertension

In this case, a possible granuloma seen on the liver biopsy suggests a granulomatous disease. This would indicate that the probable answer is sarcoidosis, TB, or berylliosis (which mimics sarcoidosis). Berylliosis should come to mind considering the patient's previous employment in the aerospace and atomic industries. Other relevant occupational exposures include the early manufacture of fluorescent lightbulbs or golf-club heads. TB can cause both granuloma and fibrosis, but is unlikely as the patient is otherwise well and afebrile. The patient's age and the fact that he is male should not let you be put off from the diagnosis. The second part of the question is easy if you have got the first part right. *Do not* leave any blank spaces: the examination is not negatively marked.

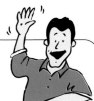

A7
a) Diagnosis
Sarcoidosis
Berylliosis
(TB)

b) Investigations
CT scan of the chest
Mediastinoscopy with lymph node biopsy

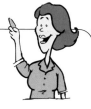

Q8

A 23-year-old woman presents to respiratory outpatients with wheeze, nocturnal cough, and shortness of breath over the last 6 months. She has also had two episodes of haemoptysis within the last 3 weeks. On both occasions she attended the casualty department, was told that she had a chest infection and was discharged with antibiotics. As a child, she had severe atopic eczema until the age of 5 years. She had the usual childhood vaccinations against measles, mumps, rubella, and whooping cough. Apart from the recent chest infections, she has otherwise been extremely well. There is a family history of atopy and her brother is a severe asthmatic. She smokes 10 cigarettes per day and works as a legal secretary in the city. She is also a keen sportswoman and until 6 months previously was in the university 100 m running team, but she now gets breathless even on mild exertion. She has only travelled to France in recent years, where she was pleased to see the French team beaten at rugby. (In this respect, then, quite normal.) A chest X-ray (CXR) taken from her casualty admission shows a shadow in the right mid-zone. A repeat CXR in the clinic shows clearing of the first shadow, but with a suspicion of another shadow in the left lower zone. Examination shows few physical signs except for some expiratory wheeze.

INVESTIGATIONS	RESULTS
Lung function tests	FEV$_1$ 1.6 l
	FVC 3.0 l
	PEFR 200 l/min
CT chest scan	Proximal bronchiectasis
FBC	Hb 10.6 g/dl
	WCC 6.2 x 10^9/l (75% neutrophils
	& 10% lymphocytes)
	Platelets 154 x 10^9/l
Urinalysis and electrolytes	Normal
Stool culture	Negative
Ca^{2+}	Normal
ACE	Normal
IgG	10 g/dl (N 10–15)
Sputum culture	Negative

ACE: angiotensin converting enzyme; FEV$_1$: forced expiratory volume in 1 second; FVC: forced vital capacity; PEFR: peak expiratory flow rate; WCC: white blood cell count. Figures in parentheses indicate normal ranges.

a) What is the most likely diagnosis?

b) Give two tests to confirm your diagnosis.

c) What would be the most appropriate treatment?

Again this should be a straightforward question if you have followed the principles given in the text so far. Do not look at the lists below but, on your own, try to decide which are the key findings that are always pathological and for which there are a limited list of causes. Write a list of these causes. Which diagnosis appears on both lists? This is likely to be the answer.

Don't turn over! (Cheat!)

Your list here...

The two lists you should have produced are for the causes of eosinophilia and proximal bronchiectasis. Here are the lists you ought to remember:

CAUSES OF EOSINOPHILIA

Skins:
Rheumatoid arthritis with cutaneous manifestations
Dermatitis herpetiformis
Scabies
Atopic eczema

Immune:
Asthma
Atopy
Any drug reactions

Neoplastic:
Hodgkin's lymphomas
Acute lymphoblastic lymphoma
All solid malignancies

Pulmonary:
Increases in sputum and peripheral blood eosinophil counts are caused by:
- allergic bronchopulmonary aspergillosis (asthma, cough, sputum plugs, proximal bronchiectasis)
- Löffler's syndrome (cough, fever, yellow sputum, malaise, fluffy X-ray infiltrates)
- tropical eosinophilia (microfilaraemia, ascariasis, ankylostomiasis, toxocariasis, strongyloidiasis)
- drug reactions (co-trimoxazole, busulphan, methotrexate, nitrofurantoin, or anything at all!)
- Churg–Strauss syndrome (small/medium-vessel vasculitis, asthma, eosinophilia)
- adult asthma

Infective:
Nematodes – roundworms (e.g. *Toxocara*, *Ascaris lumbricoides*)
Cestodes – tapeworms (e.g. *Echinococcus*)
hookworms
Trematodes – flukes
Schistosoma and other parasites
Whipple's disease

Remember that Churg–Strauss syndrome often has gut involvement, with diarrhoea and gut ulceration. In addition, there is often skin involvement, glomerulonephritis, and mononeuritis multiplex.

Causes of bronchiectasis (TACKY HI^{2}P)

- Post TB
- Aspergillosis
- Cystic fibrosis/bronchial compression
- Kartagener's syndrome (dysmotile cilia with situs inversus and infertility)
- Yellow nail syndrome
- Hypogammaglobulinaemia
- Idiopathic
- Inhalation of foreign body
- Post-childhood infection (whooping cough/pertussis, measles)

Note:

- Examiners seem to love Kartagener's syndrome: if there is the slightest hint of sinusitis, quiet heart sounds (dextrocardia), or infertility, it should be considered.
- α_1-antitrypsin deficiency can cause bronchiectasis but is better recognised for emphysema, chronic liver disease, or hepatocellular carcinoma. Diagnosis is made by serum electrophoresis.

The combination of eosinophilia and bronchiectasis has therefore led you immediately to the diagnosis. It couldn't be easier, could it? In terms of the tests to confirm your diagnoses, you will learn these answers from our book and others.

A8

a) **Diagnosis**
   Allergic bronchopulmonary aspergillosis (allergic asthma)

b) **Investigations**
   Serum IgE levels of *Aspergillus*
   Skin prick testing for *Aspergillus*
   Radioallergosorbent test (RAST)

c) **Treatment**
   These patients should be given prednisolone at an initial dose of 30 mg daily, which readily reduces the pulmonary infiltrate. Frequent episodes of this disease can be prevented by steroid treatment, but unfortunately high doses are required (10–15 mg/day).

ADDITIONAL BITS: ASPERGILLUS

Much confusion underlies *Aspergillus*. The organism:

- can colonise a lung cavity as an aspergilloma (causing cough, haemoptysis, and fever, as any lung infection)
- may invade through the lung interstitium and then disseminate around the body
- may asymptomatically colonise the lung, or may establish an allergic response causing asthma, cough, and the production of plugs of yellow eosinophilic sputum

The prick test or RAST is positive in the case of an allergic response, but not in the case of the other causes. Here is a short summary:

PROBLEM	FEATURES	PRICK TEST	PRECIPITINS/CULTURE
Colonisation	Frequently asymptomatic	−	
Aspergilloma	Cough, haemoptysis, fever	−	+
Invasive	Solely in the immuno-suppressed patients, often spreads around the body	+/−	+/−
Asthma	May be occupational	+	+
ABPA	Asthma, cough, sputum plugging. Patchy infiltrates on CXR, may show bronchiectasis	+	+ Raised IgE

ABPA: allergic broncho–pulmonary aspergillosis.

ANOTHER QUICK JOKE

A doctor arrives in clinic with a rectal thermometer behind his ear. One of the nurses points this out. "Damn!" he says, "Who the hell has got my pen?"

ADDITIONAL BITS: PLEURAL EFFUSIONS

The causes should be clear if you construct your usual 'surgical sieve'. You should always have your own sieve. Remember – our favourite is 'TIE HIM IN' to which we add a few 'can-do-anything' checks (syphilis, hypothyroidism and hyperthyroidism, sarcoidosis and amyloidosis), and a system review (think of anything that can affect, for example, the respiratory system, CNS, or gastrointestinal systems). Ensure that you remember this sieve. If you cannot, revise it (pages 13–14).

Use the sieve, and apply it to transudates and exudates in turn:

Trauma _____

Infection _____

Endocrine _____

Haematology _____

Iatrogenic _____

Metabolic _____

Idiopathic _____

Neoplastic _____

TB _____

Syphilis _____

Amyloidosis _____

Sarcoidosis _____

Autoimmune _____

Systems review _____

The ones people often miss are:

Transudates

- congestive heart failure
- nephrosis
- cirrhosis
- protein-losing enteropathy
- peritoneal dialysis

Exudates

- infection (pneumonia, TB)
- mesothelioma, local malignancy
- pulmonary embolus
- uraemia
- hypothyroidism
- subphrenic abscess
- yellow nail syndrome (NB: bronchiectasis)
- Meigs's syndrome (+ benign ovarian fibroma or thecoma +/− ascites)
- pancreatitis
- connective tissue diseases (systemic lupus erythematosus [SLE], RA)
- local trauma

Note: classically a protein concentration of less than 3 g/dl has been used to distinguish a transudate from an exudate. However, better still, the effusion is an exudate if it meets one or more of Light's criteria: ratio of pleural to serum protein levels >0.5; ratio of pleural to serum lactate dehydrogenase (LDH) levels >0.6; or pleural fluid LDH level >two-thirds the upper limit for serum LDH levels. Alternatively, a serum/pleural albumin concentration of <1.2 g/dl indicates exudation.

Assessment of a pleural effusion thus requires:

- cell count with differential, total protein level, glucose level, LDH level, amylase level, and pH (provides important prognostic information in tumours)
- cytological analysis
- Gram staining, auramine/ZN(Ziehl–Neelsen)/acid-fast bacilli staining, fungal staining (India ink/cryptococcal antigen), culture, and sensitivity testing for aerobic and anaerobic organisms and fungi
- determinations of simultaneous serum total protein, albumin, glucose, LDH, and amylase levels

Two last lists now.

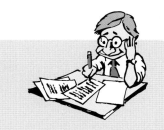

> **Cavitating lesions in the lung**
>
> *Cancers* cause cavities, so can TB*
> *Wegener's, rheumatoid**, also PE*
> *Think of the 'oses' of which there are three*
> *Also of abscesses, klebsielli*
>
> The three 'oses': histoplasmosis, coccidioidomycosis, and aspergillosis
> Abscesses (think staphylococcal, Klebsiella, amoebic, aspiration)
>
> *Small cell lung cancer; **progressive massive fibrosis/rheumatoid nodules associated with RA;
>   PE: pulmonary embolism; Wegener's: Wegener's granulomatosis

Mass lesions in the lung

Work out your own way of remembering these lists.

Single well-rounded large opacities are due to:

Neoplasms: primary malignant or metastatic (may have spiculation or cavitation)
            hamartomas (may have popcorn calcification)

Infections: bacterial; abscesses
            tuberculoma (may have calcification or satellite shadowing)
            fungal; mycetoma
            parasitic; hydatid cyst

Vascularities: arteriovenous malformations
            haematoma (post-traumatic)

Multiple well-rounded large opacities are due, in particular, to:

- sarcoidosis
- metastases
- hydatid
- abscesses or septic emboli

Multiple small (<5 mm) opacities are usually suggestive of:

- miliary TB
- sarcoidosis
- pneumoconioses
- interstitial fibrosis/alveolitis (see above)

Localised radiolucencies are due to:

- cavitation in an abscess/carcinoma/TB
- bullae
- pneumatoceles (think of cystic fibrosis)
- cystic bronchiectasis

Sarcoidosis seems to arise frequently in membership assessment, and especially in respiratory cases. Remember that it can cause lymphadenopathy and hepatosplenomegaly (and thus can mimic lymphoma). It may produce a rise in gamma-globulins, β-cells, total lymphocyte count, and serum ACE.

The space below is left blank for you to work out your own 'memory trick' for the list.

Your memory trick

Before moving on to the next chapter...

- What are the features of Horner's syndrome and its causes?
- What are the causes of papilloedema? polycythaemia? optic atrophy?
- What are the causes of choroidoretinitis? retinitis pigmentosa?
- Write down the 'BHL' list

4

METABOLLOCKS

THE METABOLIC MRCP LISTS

Abnormal biochemical findings feature heavily in the MRCP examination. Sometimes, the finding is solitary, such as hypercalcaemia. At other times, you might be expected to recognise a pattern, such as hypokalaemic alkalosis. We have produced an extensive chapter here for two reasons. Firstly, questions are common. Secondly, these issues tend not to be well addressed in other books.

Of all the abnormal biochemical findings seen, the most common are of calcium levels, and, in particular, high calcium.

IN A NUTSHELL

Remember that the calcium pool in the blood comes from gut absorption, renal calcium reabsorption, and bone resorption. Control of calcium levels requires normal renal, bone and gut function, and three normally functioning hormone systems:

1) **parathyroid hormone (PTH)**   **increases plasma calcium**

  increases renal tubular resorption

  increases osteoclast activity (bone resorption)

  increases renal conversion of 25-hydroxy-vitamin D to 1,25-dihydroxy-vitamin D

  and decreases plasma phosphate

  decreases renal phosphate reabsorption

  increases osteoclast activity with release of phosphate from bone

2) **vitamin D**   **increases plasma calcium**

  increases renal tubular reabsorption

  increases gut reabsorption

  increases osteoclast activity (bone resorption)

  increases plasma phosphate

  increases renal phosphate reabsorption

3) **hormones that broadly affect 'growth' also raise blood calcium:**
   e.g. growth hormone excess, oestrogen excess, thyrotoxicosis, excess steroids

Causes of hypercalcaemia

Abnormal control

- excess PTH:
    - primary and tertiary hyperparathyroidism
    - multiple endocrine neoplasias (MEN) I/II
    - ectopic PTH/PTH-related protein (PTHrP) (e.g. from oat cell carcinoma of the lung)
- vitamin D toxicity
- high hormone levels COAT:
    - Cushing's disease/Addison's disease
    - oestrogen excess
    - acromegaly
    - thyrotoxicosis

Bone destruction/resorption

- metastatic malignancy: the tumours that most commonly metastasise to bone are 'the 5 bs': bronchus, breast, byroid, brostate, and bidney
- myeloma and lymphoma

Five are MIIIST from the lists

- Milk-alkali syndrome
- Iatrogenic (lithium, thiazides), Idiopathic Infantile (supravalvular aortic stenosis, elfin facies)
- Sarcoid* (phosphate often normal)
- Tuberculosis (TB)* (and leprosy)

* Granulomas in general may raise calcium levels. Thus, other causes include histoplasmosis, coccidioidomycosis, and Wegener's granulomatosis.

Hypocalcaemia ...

... has a more limited list of causes:

- hypoparathyroidism, parathyroid gland excision, and pseudohypoparathyroidism
- low vitamin D levels: remember low fat diet, or malabsorption. The four fat-soluble vitamins are A, D, E, and K
- malabsorption syndromes
- chronic renal failure: tubules are resistant to hormone action resulting in low calcium and high phosphate levels. Compensatory high calcium production can lead to metastatic soft-tissue calcification
- acute pancreatitis: calcium is sequestered as 'soaps'
- rhabdomyolysis

Q9 A 52-year-old man presents with general lethargy and weakness over the past 3 weeks. He has never had any previous illnesses except for typhoid fever 3 years ago when he visited India with his wife. He has recently divorced and lives with his eldest son, who is a breeder of rare guinea fowl. He is a smoker of 20 cigarettes per day and drinks "15 pints of lager per week with the occasional whisky". He has also noticed that he has developed lower back pain. He denies any neurological symptoms in his legs. Around the same time that the back pain started he felt that he was more thirsty than usual. He has been passing urine more frequently than normal but has not suffered from any episodes of urinary or faecal incontinence.

On examination he looks well. His blood pressure is 118/68 mm/Hg. He has mild tenderness to palpation in his lumbar spine with limited straight leg raising. His neurological examination is normal and, in particular, his reflexes are normal and his plantar response is downgoing. Otherwise the examination was unremarkable.

INVESTIGATIONS	RESULTS
Plasma sodium	132 mmol/l
Plasma potassium	4.3 mmol/l
Plasma urea	15.1 mmol/l
Plasma creatinine	197 μmol/l
Liver function tests	Normal
Plasma glucose	5.4 mmol/l
Serum calcium	3.69 mmol/l
Serum albumin	39 g/l
Serum phosphate	1.3 mmol/l
Parathyroid hormone	Normal
Serum prostate specific antigen	Normal
Prostatic biopsy	Normal
Haemoglobin	8.9 g/dl
White cell count	3.3 x 10^9/l
Platelets	138 x 10^9/l
Chest X-ray	Normal
MRI lumbar spine	Normal

MRI: magnetic resonance imaging.

a) What is the most likely diagnosis?

_____

b) What is the cause of his renal impairment?

_____

c) What five investigations would now be appropriate?

_____

_____

_____

_____

_____

This is one of the classic membership examination questions and can appear in any part of the written examination. In this case, the points to be aware of are the presence of hypocalcaemia, renal impairment and anaemia. There are long lists of the causes of anaemia and renal failure, but the key word here is long. You haven't time to write a list of all the causes of acute renal failure or anaemia. Therefore, stick to your list of causes of hypercalcaemia. Revise it here:

HYPOCALCAEMIA ...

Complete the lists:

Abnormal control

1) _____

2) _____

3) _____

Bone destruction/resorption

1) _____

2) _____

3) _____

Five MIIIST from the lists

1) _____

2) _____

3) _____

4) _____

5) _____

Hyperparathyroidism is unlikely, as the PTH level is normal. In the context of such a high calcium level, the PTH should be suppressed; however, this relationship is blunted in renal failure. Cushing's disease is unlikely given the normal blood pressure, normal glucose and electrolytes, and absence of other signs. Sarcoidosis can cause hypercalcaemia and renal failure, and you would get points for this suggestion. One might argue that TB with renal involvement might do the same. However, the patient is afebrile with no nodes. This, together with the normal chest X-ray, makes these less likely. In addition, these diseases are associated with milder hypercalcaemia (generally) than this patient has. This, therefore, leaves malignancy, possibly prostatic carcinoma (perhaps with renal tract obstruction) or myeloma. As the prostate specific antigen (PSA) level is normal, myeloma is the likely cause.

Get used to this sort of process. If you have more than one finding with more than one list, then cross-reference them. If you have one list, then go through weeding out the 'impossible', and then the 'less likely'. This ought to leave one clear favourite in the field, which you should back.

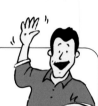

A9

a) Most likely diagnosis
Multiple myeloma

b) Cause of renal impairment
Hypercalcaemia
Nephrocalcinosis and urate nephropathy
Light chain/Bence Jones protein damage (kappa chains are worst at this: 'kappa kills kidneys')
Dehydration
Infection due to immunoparesis
Plasma cell infiltration of the kidney
Nonsteroidal anti-inflammatory drug (NSAID) damage (taken for the back pain)
Amyloidosis

c) Appropriate investigations
Serum electrophoresis (presence of a monoclonal band)
Serum immunoglobulins
Bence Jones protein in the urine
Skeletal survey
Bone marrow biopsy

The list of causes of renal failure in myeloma (above) is itself worth learning.

Q10

A 73-year-old man presents with a 3-month history of weight loss and the recent onset of confusion. He thinks that he might have had one episode of haemoptysis 2 days before his clinic visit. He denies other symptoms, but his wife says that he has been complaining of intermittent headaches, has appeared 'distant' over the same period of time, and has lost interest in his main pastime of gardening. (The book editors view this hobby as evidence of a *longstanding* impairment of mental function!) He gave up smoking 5 years earlier, after a 60 pack-year history. He was previously diagnosed as having mild chronic bronchitis and uses salbutamol and beclomethasone inhalers for this. On further questioning he says that he has lost his appetite. He denies any associated fevers. There is no history of recent foreign travel, although he did serve in the army during the war and was stationed in North Africa where he suffered from one episode of malaria. He denies any gastrointestinal symptoms and has never suffered with cardiac disease. He does admit to coughing up sputum most mornings and this has been worse recently.

On examination, he appears cachectic with proximal muscle wasting. He has evidence of a peripheral neuropathy, more pronounced in the arms than the legs. Fundoscopy is normal and there is no evidence of long tract, parietal, or cerebellar signs. He is in atrial fibrillation with a pulse rate of 100 beats/min. His blood pressure is 123/72 mmHg. There are no signs in the respiratory tract. Abdominal examination is unremarkable.

INVESTIGATIONS	RESULTS
Serum sodium	135 mmol/l
Serum potassium	3.6 mmol/l
Serum urea	10.8 mmol/l
Plasma creatinine	98 μmol/l
Creatinine phosphokinase	100 IU/l
Serum alkaline phosphatase	100 IU/l
Serum aspartate aminotransferase	8 IU/l
Serum alanine aminotransferase	6 IU/l
Serum calcium	2.65 mmol/l
Serum albumin	30 g/l
Parathyroid hormone	Normal
Sputum AFB	Negative x 3
Serum electrophoresis	No monoclonal bands seen
Chest X-ray	Cavitating lesion in the right midzone

AFB: acid-fast bacilli.

a) What is the most likely diagnosis?

_____

b) Give two reasons for his confusion.

_____

_____

c) What three tests would now be appropriate?

_____

_____

Even if you spotted the answer straight away, work your way through the method, and learn the lists. What are the findings that are always abnormal and for which there are limited lists of causes? Decide, and then write down the relevant lists. Which diagnosis appears on all the lists? This is the correct answer. Again, _don't look down!_

The definitively abnormal findings are hypercalcaemia, peripheral neuropathy, and a cavitating lesion in the lung. You already have a list for the causes of peripheral neuropathy. You now need lists for the causes of hypercalcaemia and of lung cavitation.

Let's first deal with the hypercalcaemia. You should have this off to a tee by now.

_____

_____

_____

_____

_____

_____

_____

_____

_____

_____

_____

You have learned the causes of peripheral neuropathy (fill in the list below to refresh your memory):

PERIPHERAL NEUROPATHY

Congenital (born unlucky): _____

Three dejected: _____

Two infected: _____

Two injected: _____

One connected: _____

_____ suspected and _____ , which just refuses to rhyme.

And here are the causes of lung cavitation ... remember the rhyme (Pants, page 61)?

CAVITATING LESIONS IN THE LUNG

- Cancers (squamous cell carcinoma)
- TB
- Wegener's granulomatosis
- Rheumatoid arthritis
- Pulmonary embolism
- Three 'oses': histoplasmosis, coccidioidomycosis and aspergillosis
- Abscesses: staphylococcal, Klebsiella, amoebiasis, and aspiration

Untreated, TB is not commonly a cause of peripheral neuropathy. If the patient was receiving treatment with isoniazid, however, then this would have been a potential diagnosis.

Vasculitis can also be associated with peripheral neuropathy, and a Wegener's-like granulomatosis might be considered, except for the hypercalcaemia. Sarcoidosis, too, might be considered as a cause of neuropathy and hypercalcaemia, but is not a cause of lung *cavitation*.

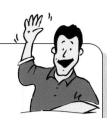

A10

a) Diagnosis
Squamous carcinoma of the bronchus

b) Reasons for confusion
Hypercalcaemia
Cerebral metastases

c) Investigations
CT scan of chest
Bronchoscopy
CT scan of the head

CT: computed tomography.

Q11

A 45-year-old woman presents to her doctor with polyuria and polydipsia. She is not diabetic and her blood sugar is normal. On further questioning she admits to having had intermittent abdominal pain for several months, accompanied by vomiting and constipation. She is very worried because her father died last year from oesophageal carcinoma and she herself has smoked 20–30 cigarettes per day since she was 16 years old. There is nothing to find on examination. Her GP arranges to see her in 1 month, and meanwhile organises a plain abdominal film and some screening blood tests.

INVESTIGATION	RESULTS
Abdominal X-ray	Evidence of bilateral nephrocalcinosis
White cell count	$8.4 \times 10^9/l$
Haemoglobin	11.7 g/dl
Platelets	$376 \times 10^9/l$
Plasma urea	8.1 mmol/l
Plasma creatinine	165 μmol/l
Plasma sodium	140 mmol/l
Plasma potassium	4.3 mmol/l
Serum calcium	2.80 mmol/l
Serum phosphate	0.70 mmol/l

a) Which is the most likely single diagnosis?

- paraneoplastic hypercalcaemia of malignancy
- primary hyperparathyroidism
- familial hypocalciuric hypercalcaemia (FHH)

b) Which would be the most helpful investigation?

- parathyroid hormone assay
- urinary cyclic adenosine monophosphate (cAMP)
- hydrocortisone suppression test
- 24-hour urinary calcium excretion
- PTHrP radioimmunoassay

A11

a) Diagnosis

The obvious abnormal feature here is hypercalcaemia. You really ought, by now, to have the table of causes 'off pat'. Of the choices given, nephrocalcinosis only occurs in primary hyperparathyroidism, so this must be the diagnosis. You might not have known this before, but you do now!

b) Test

The most helpful test is the one that excludes the other diagnoses. In this instance, it is the hydrocortisone suppression test; hydrocortisone suppresses calcium levels in other causes of hypercalcaemia, but not in primary hyperparathyroidism.

CHOROIDORETINITIS CAUSES

Find the right start square, then follow to adjacent boxes (only vertically or horizontally) to find some causes of choroidoretinitis. There are a few other words in there which are not causes. What are they? Once you have finished, look at the answers (page 107) and revise the causes (page 34).

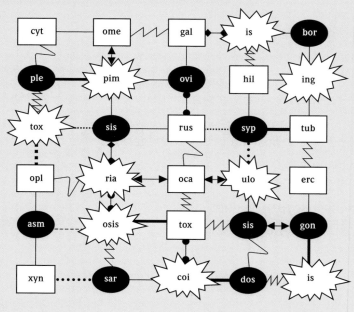

REVIEW OF POSSIBLE DIAGNOSES

Here is a quick summary of the main features of the three possible diagnoses.

PRIMARY HYPERPARATHYROIDISM	HYPERCALCAEMIA OF MALIGNANCY	FAMILIAL HYPOCALCIURIC HYPERCALCAEMIA (FHH)
80% single adenoma 10% gland hyperplasia 2% parathyroid carcinoma	Squamous cell carcinoma (lung, oesophagus) renal/breast/ovary/ pancreas/bladder/lymph	Autosomal dominant Abnormal calcium receptors
Very high PTH	High PTHrP	High/normal PTH
High calcium, low phosphate	High calcium, low phosphate	Very high calcium – stays high post parathyroidectomy
High urinary cAMP	High urinary cAMP	
High 24-hour urine calcium	High 24-hour urine calcium	Low 24-hour urine calcium
Polyuria/polydipsia	Polyuria/polydipsia	Benign/asymptomatic
Nephrocalcinosis	No nephrocalcinosis	No nephrocalcinosis
Subperiosteal erosions	Bony erosions	No bony abnormalities
Less acute onset	More acute onset	Usually found by chance
Bones, moans, stones, and abdominal groans	Symptoms and signs of primary cancer	
Associated with a hyperchloraemic metabolic acidosis	May have hypochloraemic metabolic alkalosis if much vomiting/polyuria	
Hydrocortisone suppression test doesn't suppress calcium in primary hyperparathyroidism, but does in other causes of hypercalcaemia	PTH radioimmunoassay readily differentiates between PTH and PTHrP	FHH = CaCl/CrCl <0.01 Primary PTH >0.01

CaCI: calcium clearance; cAMP: cyclic AMP; CrCI: creatine clearance; PTH: parathyroid hormone; PTHrP: parathyroid hormone–related protein.

Q 12

A young girl is seen in the endocrine clinic after referral from her GP who found her to be hypocalcaemic. She has a fairly long-standing history of intermittent diarrhoea, which has never been investigated. She was achieving well at school until last year when her family moved to London because of her mother's job. Since then her grades are not as good as they used to be. She confides in you that some of the bigger girls in her year have been bullying her, so she has been skipping the first and last lessons of the day in an attempt to try to avoid them. She has no significant past medical history other than mild asthma, which is well-controlled. She has never been hospitalised. On examination, she is a pretty girl, with a round face. You notice that on her right hand she has shortened ring and little fingers. Examination is otherwise unremarkable.

INVESTIGATIONS	RESULTS
Serum calcium	1.95 (corrected) mmol/l
Serum phosphate	1.7 mmol/l
Plasma urea	4.3 mmol/l
Plasma creatinine	121 μmol/l
Plasma sodium	137 mmol/l
Plasma potassium	3.9 mmol/l
Serum albumin	39 g/l
Iron studies	Normal
Clotting	Normal
Haemoglobin	12.6 g/dl
White cell count	5.8 x 10⁹/l
Platelets	234 x 10⁹/l

a) What is the diagnosis?

- Type I pseudohypoparathyroidism
- Type II pseudohypoparathyroidism
- Turner's syndrome
- pseudohypoparathyroidism

b) Which is the most discriminating test?

- PTH estimation
- Response to PTH infusion
- Serum magnesium
- Buccal smear

The key abnormal finding that has a limited list of causes is hypocalcaemia. List the causes now in the space below. When you have done this, they are given below to refresh your memory.

_____

_____

_____

_____

CAUSES OF HYPOCALCAEMIA

- Hypoparathyroidism and parathyroid gland excision: pseudohypoparathyroidism
- Low vitamin D levels (remember low fat diet/sunlight/absorption)
- Malabsorption syndromes
- Chronic renal failure
- Acute pancreatitis (calcium sequestered as 'soaps')
- Rhabdomyolysis

In this case, she clearly does not have acute pancreatitis/rhabdomyolysis. Chronic renal failure is excluded by the normal urea and creatinine levels. By telling you that the albumin and iron studies are normal, the examiners are trying to tell you that there is no significant malabsorption. In particular, the normal international normalised ratio (INR), which has been given in the investigations, suggests normal vitamin K levels, and hence a low likelihood of abnormal absorption of fat-soluble vitamins: with normal sunlight exposure, this makes vitamin D levels likely to be normal. She thus seems to have _pseudohypoparathyroidism_ (type I). The causes are listed in the summary table on the next page. Learn it now. From it, you should be able to figure out that the correct answer to the question is Albright's hereditary osteodystrophy (AHO), and that the most helpful investigation is the PTH infusion test. This involves taking baseline, 30-, 60-, and 90-minute urine samples for phosphate and cyclic AMP (cAMP), while giving 200 units of PTH intravenously over 10 minutes between collections; this is usually performed in a metabolic unit!

At this point, it is worth reviewing the familial hypocalcaemic/hypophosphataemic syndromes. In examinations, a patient will be presented with familial hypocalcaemia and hypophosphataemia who is symptomatic with signs and symptoms of hypocalcaemia and rickets. Although these cases are almost always presented badly the answer is invariably simple.

Low calcium and low phosphate levels (as well as rickets) must mean a defect in vitamin D metabolism. Once this is appreciated, quickly think back to vitamin D metabolism. Vitamin D is either ingested or converted from cholesterol by sunlight in the skin and further metabolised in the liver (to 25 hydroxy-cholecalciferol) and finally in the kidneys to active 1,25 dihydroxy-vitamin D. It then acts upon its intracellular receptor.

Thus, low calcium/phosphate levels are either due to poor diet or vitamin D absorption, poor sun exposure, or failure of liver/kidney metabolism or receptor function. Familial type I rickets is a failure of kidney metabolism with low 1,25-dihydroxy-vitamin D, and is easily treated with 1,25-dihydroxy-vitamin D supplementation. Familial type II rickets is a receptor defect, and is characterised by end-organ resistance. In such cases, 1,25-dihydroxy-vitamin D levels are high, and the condition is treated (though less effectively) with high doses of vitamin D and phosphate. Both of these conditions left untreated have raised PTH levels.

Do not confuse these with the X-linked hypophosphataemic rickets (X-linked dominant), which is associated with normal calcium and PTH levels, low phosphate levels, and rickets.

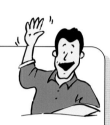

A12 a) **Diagnosis**
pseudohypoparathyroidism (Albright's hereditary osteodystrophy [AHO])

b) **Test**
PTH infusion test

REVIEW OF POSSIBLE DIAGNOSES

Here is a quick summary of the main features of the three possible diagnoses.

	TYPE I PSEUDO-HYPOPARATHYROIDISM	TYPE II PSEUDO-HYPOPARATHYRODISM	PSEUDOPSEUDO-HYPOPARATHYROIDISM	TURNER'S SYNDROME
Nature	G-protein disorder with end-organ resistance to PTH	Failure of renal response to cAMP	No abnormal pathology	XO genotype
PTH	Appropriately high	Appropriately high	Normal	Normal or slightly high
Calcium	Low	Low	Normal	Normal
Phosphate	High	High	Normal	Normal
Phenotype	Unusual, with round face and short fourth and fifth metacarpals	Normal	Unusual, as for AHO	Can be associated with short fourth and fifth metacarpals
Urine	Low urine phosphate and cAMP response to PTH infusion	Normal urine cAMP but low urine phosphate in response to PTH infusion	Normal urine cAMP and phosphate in response to PTH infusion	Normal urine cAMP and phosphate in response to PTH infusion

Turner's syndrome

Patients with Turner's syndrome (X0) have short stature, a wide carrying angle, webbed-neck, widely spaced nipples, shield-chests, and ovarian failure, which causes osteoporosis. They may also suffer autoimmune hypothyroidism/diabetes mellitus, renal dysgenesis, aortic coarctation/dissection, lymphoedema, and gonadoblastoma. X-linked recessive disorders that usually affect men include haemophilia.

Time for a quick **WORDSEARCH** over a cuppa. Find the 11 syndromes or tests bearing the discoverer's name in the grid below. They can occur diagonally, vertically and horizontally, either backwards or forwards. Write down three lines on each as you find them. These syndromes will be covered throughout the book.

A	L	B	R	I	G	H	T	S	H	J	G	Q	S	T	A	R	D	D	A
W	A	S	D	F	G	Y	T	L	L	E	D	T	B	N	J	K	L	R
A	S	D	K	R	D	E	F	G	H	S	S	G	Q	U	I	H	C	L	M
I	O	P	E	E	C	F	E	O	L	L	D	E	W	C	V	N	H	K	L
O	R	F	S	H	S	D	G	N	C	M	W	E	I	L	S	M	R	M	M
W	J	K	E	E	D	S	E	C	M	S	W	F	F	F	D	W	I	I	U
H	L	B	L	L	W	W	R	F	G	W	E	K	L	J	K	R	S	X	M
A	S	W	A	A	S	Y	U	E	O	P	H	O	D	S	U	I	T	N	E
M	W	E	S	D	D	D	C	X	I	S	W	G	O	W	L	P	M	M	D
S	S	D	E	E	S	N	M	R	R	R	D	W	V	M	K	D	A	P	S
T	W	J	F	R	H	K	L	X	F	R	A	R	K	F	D	S	S	G	E
E	E	V	N	H	D	S	W	W	B	M	N	D	E	O	F	U	L	P	I
S	S	W	E	S	G	K	R	E	E	E	H	K	M	N	E	X	K	D	I
T	E	S	E	I	G	D	N	S	G	T	L	J	N	A	F	I	G	D	H
W	A	I	D	F	V	B	D	E	S	D	H	I	W	S	H	L	E	D	R
W	P	K	P	P	F	J	Q	A	V	M	Z	S	W	J	K	W	L	Y	E
F	V	A	V	V	R	E	I	L	U	O	S	D	R	A	N	R	E	B	G
F	A	S	C	G	U	H	W	I	L	J	A	K	L	G	S	D	Q	T	A
X	C	A	S	U	J	L	F	W	E	E	G	E	W	S	D	J	F	E	R
W	O	W	P	J	W	A	S	S	S	R	A	F	R	E	S	A	J	K	D
W	P	A	B	D	H	L	S	A	W	E	H	W	A	F	A	N	H	U	Y
D	K	L	G	S	J	J	R	S	E	V	C	S	H	L	H	E	Q	U	H
C	N	G	D	S	G	H	P	S	S	Q	D	G	K	E	K	E	A	C	S
F	I	K	F	S	E	J	Q	P	G	S	H	C	Z	M	J	G	F	E	E
Y	L	F	A	N	C	O	N	I	S	R	G	E	O	H	P	O	L	E	S

Shy–Drager, Weils

Answers: Albrights, Behcets, Bernard Soulier, Chagas, Christmas, Dariers, Fanconis, Hams test, Kawasakis,

WATER, WATER EVERYWHERE...

The last question might have alarmed you by reminding you about diabetes mellitus, diabetes insipidus, and the causes of polyuria and polydipsia. Fear not! Here is all you need to know about water.

Firstly, water is the most important molecule on the planet, being the primary constituent of beer. Any other facts are superfluous.

Water overload causes dilution. Low levels of urea, sodium, and potassium together should alert you to the diagnosis. Causes are divided into the 'too much in' and 'too little out' categories.

Too much in

Causes include: psychogenic polydipsia, hypothalamic tumour (leading to excess thirst), iatrogenic (drip), and water retained in excess of salt, such as in states of oedema – congestive heart failure, cirrhosis, nephrotic oedema, and myxoedema.

Too little out

In the syndrome of inappropriate antidiuretic hormone secretion (SIADH), plasma osmolality is low, but urine osmolality is higher than that of plasma. Urinary sodium excretion may also be raised. Sorry (in advance) for the bad pun, but the causes of SIADH are 'CCCP', as *there ain't no water 'Russian' out!*

Chest:	infections (abscess, effusions, pneumonia, TB) tumours (small cell carcinoma especially)
Cerebral:	infections (abscess, meningitis, TB) tumours (cerebral)
Cancers:	lung and other sites rarely, such as pancreas
Ps:	**p**leural effusions, **p**ancreatitis, **p**orphyria, and **p**ills CCCAN (**c**arbamazepine, **c**hlorpropamide, **c**lofibrate, **a**ntipsychotics, **N**SAIDs)

Pure salt depletion is unusual as a cause of hyponatraemia, but can occur with diarrhoea/vomiting if adequate water intake is sustained. Beware pseudohyponatraemia, when cholesterol and fat levels in the blood take up space in the sample volume, and lead to erroneous assessment of serum sodium. This occurs in nephrotic syndrome and in ketoacidosis.

... AND NOT A DROP TO DRINK

Diabetes insipidus (DI)

This is due to lack of ADH action, which may be due to:

- low production:
  anything destroying posterior pituitary function: hypothalamic damage, craniopharyngioma, pituitary stalk damage (e.g. Sheehan's syndrome of pituitary stalk infarction complicating post-partum haemorrhagic shock), pituitary tumours, basal meningitis (particularly tuberculous meningitis), sarcoidosis (work your way through your surgical sieve)

- resistance to action:
  drugs: such as lithium, or amphotericin therapy
  electrolytes: prolonged hypercalcaemia, hypokalaemia or hyponatraemia, or distal tubular disease
  inherited: nephrogenic DI (X-linked)

Note: hypoadrenalism also prevents the normal concentration of urine.

Answers to causes of erythema nodosum (page 150): sarcoidosis, TB, the pill, sulphonamides, bromides, iodides, streptococci, IBD, histoplasmosis, blastomycosis (and horse and mules).

Q 13

A 29-year-old man presents to his GP with polydipsia and polyuria. He drinks 8–10 pints of water daily and wakes several times in the night to pass water and because of thirst. He is afebrile and has lost no body mass. His mother, who is of Antiguan origin, has poorly controlled diabetes but does not yet take insulin. His father is hypertensive and there is no other relevant family history. The patient works in the music industry and has no past history of note. Clinical examination is unremarkable.

GP PRELIMINARY INVESTIGATIONS	RESULTS
BM (blood sugar)	4.2
Urine dipstick	No glucose, protein, or blood
	Specific gravity low

ENDOCRINE CLINIC INVESTIGATIONS	ENDOCRINE CLINIC RESULTS
Plasma sodium	141 mmol/l
Plasma potassium	3.7 mmol/l
Plasma urea	8.0 mmol/l
Serum albumin	40 g/l
Serum calcium	2.3 mmol/l
Plasma glucose	4.5 mmol/l
Plasma osmolality	293 mOsmol/l
Urine osmolality	80 mOsmol/l
Water deprivation test	Posm at 6 hours = 308 mOsmol/l
	Uosm at 6 hours = 100 mOsmol/l
	Posm after DDAVP = 290 mOsmol/l
	Uosm after DDAVP = 900 mOsmol/l
Chest X-ray	Bilateral hilar lymphadenopathy, mild
	reticular shadowing in apical lung fields

DDAVP: 1-deamino-8-D-arginine vasopressin; Posm: plasma osmolality; Uosm: urine osmolality.

a) **What is the cause of this man's symptoms?**

b) **What would you expect to find on transbronchial biopsy?**

c) **What is the underlying diagnosis?**

The key abnormal findings here are:
- cranial diabetes insipidus
- bilateral hilar lymphadenopathy (BHL)

We have already been through the causes of BHL. Jot them down here.

Now check that you got them all:

- sarcoidosis and TB
- lymphoma and cancers
- Churg–Strauss syndrome, phenytoin treatment, extrinsic allergic alveolitis, pneumoconiosis (especially berylliosis), cystic fibrosis, and HIV

The patient has nothing at all to suggest Churg–Strauss syndrome or HIV, he has not been exposed to beryllium, and he is not receiving phenytoin treatment. The absence of systemic features or findings is against TB, lymphoma, or other malignancy. Thus, the likeliest diagnosis is of sarcoidosis.

A13

a) Symptom cause
Cranial diabetes insipidus secondary to granulomatous pituitary infiltration

b) Transbronchial biopsy findings
Noncaseating granulomata (granuloma on its own here is not enough to get full marks)

c) Underlying diagnosis
Sarcoidosis

Treatment

The treatment of choice for cranial DI is administration of synthetic vasopressin. The most convenient route of administration is intranasally, usually 2–3 times daily.

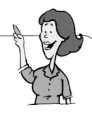

Q14

A 25-year-old man is admitted to casualty following a road traffic accident, during which he briefly lost consciousness. He had lost control of the vehicle and tells you that he had taken Ecstasy and "two beers" that night. He is found to have a closed fracture of his left tibia and fibula. Despite the fact that the orthopaedic senior house officer (SHO) is keen to discharge the patient with a Tubigrip, he is admitted for surgical treatment under general anaesthesia. Afterwards, he complains of slight headache, and coryza with a runny nose. He was treated for non-Hodgkin's lymphoma at the age of 18 years, and smokes 15 cigarettes per day. He takes occasional cocaine on Saturday nights. Some 36 hours postoperatively, physicians are asked to see him, as he appears to have developed an acute confusional state. The nurses report that he has oliguria. His blood tests from that morning are as follows.

Investigation	Results
Plasma sodium	120 mmol/l
Plasma urea	2.8 mmol/l
Plasma potassium	3.2 mmol/l
Plasma creatinine	45 μmol/l
Plasma glucose	5.2 mmol/l

a) **Suggest two reasons for the above results.**

b) **What immediate management step would you take?**

This poor fellow has severe hyponatraemia following surgery. The temptation is immediately to blame the orthopaedic consultant for his fluid management. *In general, this is a good idea and is to be encouraged. Please speak slowly, however, so that they can keep up. Wave a £20 note intermittently to keep their attention.*

However, you must remember that the patient has also had a closed head injury. The fact that he is oliguric suggests that he might be suffering from SIADH.

Finally, Ecstasy overdose can lead to a variety of metabolic abnormalities, as can excessive drinking of fluids whilst taking it. However, probably too much time has lapsed for these effects to be responsible for the patient's symptoms.

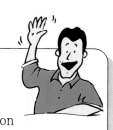

A14 **a) Reasons for the results**
Syndrome of inappropriate ADH secretion (SIADH)
following head injury
Excess intravenous dextrose resulting in plasma dilution

b) Immediate management
Fluid restriction

Another favourite scenario in the examination is that under different circumstances trauma may lead to central DI due to damage to the posterior pituitary.

HYPONATRAEMIA

It is useful to think of hyponatraemia in terms of a patient's fluid balance, as below.

OEDEMATOUS	NORMAL FLUID BALANCE	DEHYDRATED
Excess body water >excess sodium	Excess body water + normal body sodium	Sodium loss >water loss
Examples	Examples	Examples
• CHF	• SIADH (all causes)	• Adrenal insufficiency
• Cirrhosis	• Pseudohyponatraemia	• GI losses (diarrhoea and
• Nephrotic syndrome	• (hyperglycaemia,	vomiting, fistula)
• Myxoedema	hyperlipidaemia, myeloma)	• Renal losses (diuretics,
	• Psychogenic polydipsia	osmotic diuresis, renal
		tubular disease)

CHF: congestive heart failure; GI: gastrointestinal.

Remember, too, that:

$$\text{Calculated plasma osmolality} = 2(Na + K) + \text{urea} + \text{glucose}$$

You can use this trick in casualty. Calculate the osmolality, then ask the laboratory to measure it. They are usually happier to do this than to measure a blood alcohol level. Work out the difference between the calculated and real measurements. This difference must be ascribed to some metabolically active agent in the blood. If the patient has been drinking, you can assume that this substance is alcohol. As 1 mmol of alcohol is responsible for 1 mOsmol, you can now calculate the mmol/L of alcohol. Knowing the relative molecular mass of alcohol (from its formula C_2H_5OH) you can calculate the number of mg/dl!

Potassium page

Potassium and pH

Hydrogen and potassium ions can be considered to compete for cellular handling. Thus, as potassium levels rise, fewer hydrogen ions can enter into cells, and plasma hydrogen levels rise. At the renal tubule, excess potassium also limits hydrogen excretion. Thus, primary hyperkalaemia is associated with acidosis (hyperkalaemic acidosis), and primary potassium depletion with alkalosis (hypokalaemic alkalosis). The same association of potassium and hydrogen is seen in primary metabolic acidosis and alkalosis. Thus, hypokalaemic alkalosis is seen in situations of excess potassium loss. Hypokalaemic acidosis, on the other hand, needs a loss of both bicarbonate and potassium. Draw up a list of causes of hypokalaemic alkalosis and hypokalaemic acidosis; then check it against the list below.

and remember....

... glucocorticoids and mineralocorticoids are sodium sparing and potassium wasting.

Hypokalaemic alkalosis	Hypokalaemic acidosis
'Steroid hormones GIVe VILe Diuresis'	'PARADE'
Steroid: Conn's syndrome, Cushing's disease, corticosteroid treatment, phaeochromocytoma, liquorice and carbenoxolone **GI:** Vomiting **VI**llous adenoma, **L**axative **D**iuretics (e.g. thiazides)	**P**artially-treated diabetic ketoacidosis (already acid: insulin drives potassium into cells) **A**cetazolamide **R**enal tubular **A**cidosis (type I = proximal, type II = distal) **D**iarrhoea + hypovolaemic shock **E**nteric (ureterosigmoidostomy or biliary/pancreatic fistula leading to bicarbonate loss: vipoma with MEN I)

MEN: multiple endocrine neoplasia.

Remember the inherited tubulopathies

Defects in the loop of Henle channels, which actively reabsorb sodium from the distal convoluted tubule, lead to excessive distal convoluted tubule salt loading and eventually salt loss (e.g. in Bartter's or Gitelman syndrome). The result is biochemically similar to blockade from loop diuretics: polyuria, hypokalaemic alkalosis, hypocalcaemia, and high salt secretion are seen. For various reasons (led by high angiotensin II levels), they also have growth inhibition and intellectual retardation. They may be dysmorphic or have sensorineural hearing loss. *Thus, you might* **say** *that the patient with Bartter's syndrome is strangely 'short' on IQ, potassium, sodium, and calcium, but he might not hear you!*

Treatment includes sodium, potassium, calcium, and magnesium supplementation, use of spironolactone (an aldosterone antagonist), amiloride, and angiotensin converting enzyme (ACE) inhibitors. Growth hormone (GH) is used to treat short stature.

In addition, prolonged hypokalaemia is a cause of polyuria and polydipsia. Other causes to bear in mind are:

- prolonged hypercalcaemia
- diabetes mellitus and diabetes insipidus
- recovery phase of acute tubular necrosis, or after release of obstruction
- psychogenic polydipsia
- chronic renal impairment

Now three quick questions to keep you going . . .

Q 15

A 55-year-old man presents to casualty with lethargy, polyuria, and polydipsia. He finds this distressing as he is unable to go ballroom dancing, which he usually does at the weekends. He has been widowed for the last 18 months and takes no regular medication. His clinical examination is unremarkable other than his blood pressure which is 175/105 mm Hg. The results of a blood test are shown below.

INVESTIGATION	RESULT
Plasma sodium	148 mmol/l
Plasma bicarbonate	37 mmol/l
Serum calcium	2.30 mmol/l
Plasma potassium	2.5 mmol/l
Plasma chloride	98 mmol/l
Serum albumin	38 g/l
Plasma creatinine	100 μmol/l
Plasma glucose	5.2 mmol/l

a) What is the underlying diagnosis?

b) Give two biochemical and two radiological tests to confirm the diagnosis.

c) Give two radiological tests to confirm the diagnosis.

A15

a) **Diagnosis**

The patient has a hypokalaemic alkalosis. He is also hypertensive. Thus, the diagnosis is Conn's syndrome

b) **Biochemical tests**

24-hour urine potassium excretion (inappropriately high for serum potassium)

Serum aldosterone (elevated and not suppressible)

Plasma renin (reduced due to negative feedback from high aldosterone)

c) **Radiological tests**

CT abdomen

Bilateral adrenal vein sampling (differentiates unilateral aldosterone-producing adenoma from bilateral adrenal hyperplasia)

Note: If there is hypokalaemic/hypochloraemic alkalosis, think vomiting/gastric outlet obstruction.

CONN'S SYNDROME

This results from a primary excess of mineralocorticoids, causing sodium retention and potassium loss. However, the sodium retention causes hyperosmolality, and thus increased ADH secretion and volume expansion. There is a hypokalaemic alkalosis with low bicarbonate levels, low/normal or only slightly elevated sodium levels, and hypertension.

POLYURIA AND POLYDIPSIA

The patient also complained of polyuria and polydipsia. In this case, the biochemical tests showed the patient to be hypokalaemic. However, in the absence of any other data, the causes of polyuria and polydipsia, are useful to know, and are (as listed earlier):

- hypokalaemia
- hypercalcaemia
- diabetes mellitus
- diabetes insipidus
- recovering acute tubular necrosis, or chronic renal failure
- psychogenic polydipsia

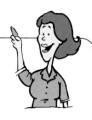

Q16 A 45-year-old woman presents to surgeons with abdominal pain, weight loss, and malaise. Apart from mild hypothyroidism she has otherwise been well. On examination she appears somewhat dehydrated.

INVESTIGATION	RESULT
Pulse	110 beats/min
Blood pressure	90/45 mm Hg
Temperature	36.6°C
Abdominal examination	Generalised abdominal tenderness
Urinalysis	Normal
Plasma sodium	125 mmol/l
Plasma potassium	6.9 mmol/l
Plasma urea	16 mmol/l
Plasma bicarbonate	15 mmol/l

a) **What is the diagnosis?**

b) **How could this be confirmed quickly?**

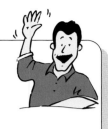

A16 **a) Diagnosis**
The obvious feature here is a hyperkalaemic acidosis.
The patient also has abdominal pain and hypotension.
Thus, the diagnosis is Addison's disease.

b) Quick test
The test is a short tetracosactrin (ACTH: adrenocorticotrophic
hormone) test followed by a therapeutic trial of steroids.

ADDISON'S DISEASE

This is caused by adrenal failure. Patients may be tanned, with scar/palmar crease/buccal pigmentation. Acute cortisol deficiency causes nausea and vomiting, general malaise, and weight loss. This compounds the renal sodium loss due to adrenal hormone deficiency, and hyponatraemia, hypotension, uraemia, and hyperkalaemic acidosis are seen. A normal cortisol level at any time of day excludes the diagnosis, as does a normal short tetracosactrin test (tetracosactrin 250 μg i.m. raises cortisol levels by >200 nmol/l to >550 nmol/l), a 5-hour test (tetracosactrin 1 mg i.m.: cortisol levels are 600–1300 nmol/l at 1 hour and 1000–1800 nmol/l at 5 hours), or a 3-day test (tetracosactrin 1 mg daily: check levels daily at 5 hours; a rising response over 3 days suggests a chronic lack of adrenocorticotrophic hormone [ACTH]).

Causes of Addison's disease

You should know these. Construct a quick list here from your surgical sieve:

_____

_____

_____

_____

_____

_____

_____

_____

_____

_____

_____

Our list

Remember:

Congenital: Rare – congenital adrenal hyperplasia is the most common cause

Acquired:

T:

I: TB, fungi (including *Cryptococcus*, coccidioidomycosis, histoplasmosis), *Neisseria meningitidis* (Waterhouse–Frederichsen syndrome)

E: H: I: M:

I: Drugs such as rifampicin, phenytoin, carbamazepine

N: Metastases

… and autoimmune adrenal failure

Note: patients must be warned to increase their dose of maintenance steroids during intercurrent infection and with treatment with enzyme inducers, such as rifampicin; in examinations beware of a patient with Addison's disease who is being treated for TB.

Quiz Spot!

Q: Polycythaemia rubra vera, myelofibrosis, and myeloproliferative disorders cause a raised leucocyte alkaline phosphatase. What else does?

A: Hodgkin's

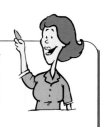

Q 17

An 11-year-old girl is admitted with a history of abdominal pain, vomiting, and malaise. She has no previous history of any illnesses. Clinical examination reveals only mild abdominal tenderness.

INVESTIGATIONS	RESULTS
Pulse	110 beats/min
Blood pressure	95/65 mm Hg
Temperature	36.8°C
Plasma sodium	128 mmol/l
Plasma potassium	6.8 mmol/l
Plasma urea	12 mmol/l
Plasma bicarbonate	7 mmol/l

a) What is the diagnosis?

b) What is your immediate management, after confirmation of your suspicions?

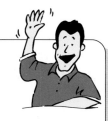

A17

a) **Diagnosis**

This is a classic MRCP examination case of diabetic ketoacidosis. Often, the sodium will be presented as much lower, due to pseudohyponatraemia from high blood lipid/cholesterol levels

b) **Immediate management**

After confirming the diagnosis with a blood glucose and urinalysis, aggressive normal saline rehydration is the key. Only when the patient has intravenous fluids being infused should a sliding scale of insulin be started and the cause of this complication be addressed

MORE ABOUT ADDISON'S DISEASE

Why is the diagnosis in this case also not Addison's disease? This is because Addison's disease rarely causes such a severe metabolic acidosis as diabetic ketoacidosis. The bicarbonate level in Addison's disease rarely falls below 15 mmol/l.

However, it is worth remembering that Addison's disease can present in a patient with diabetes. This association is known as Schmidt's syndrome.

DID YOU KNOW...

... that phaeochromocytomas cause hyperkalaemia and can be identified on ultrasound/ MRI/CT, or using MIBG (meta-iodobenzylguanidine) scanning?

... that both Conn's syndrome and hyperosmolar nonketotic hyperglycaemia cause low potassium and high sodium levels?

In a nutshell...

...remember the following equations:

1) $H^+ + HCO_3^- \leftrightharpoons H_2CO_3 \leftrightharpoons H_2O + CO_2$

2) $pH \propto \dfrac{\log[HCO_3^-]}{pCO_2}$

Metabolic acidosis

Metabolic acidosis adds hydrogen ions, which lower bicarbonate concentration and pH. Compensation is by increased respiratory drive, blowing off carbon dioxide, and normalising pH (equation 2).

Metabolic alkalosis

Metabolic alkalosis loses hydrogen ions. The first equation therefore moves from right to left, and bicarbonate concentration and pH rise (equation 2). Compensation is by retaining carbon dioxide (equation 2).

Respiratory acidosis

Respiratory acidosis gains CO_2, causing bicarbonate concentration and hydrogen concentration to rise, and the pH falls. Compensation is by retaining bicarbonate (equation 2).

Think:

- respiratory depression (raised intracranial pressure, drugs such as opioids and barbiturates, and overdoses)

- neuromuscular disease (neuropathy such as Guillain–Barré syndrome, motor neurone disease), myopathy

- skeletal disease (thoracic cage abnormalities: kyphoscoliosis and ankylosing spondylitis)

Respiratory alkalosis

Respiratory alkalosis loses carbon dioxide, equation 1 moves from left to right, and hydrogen and bicarbonate concentrations and pH fall. Compensation is by losing bicarbonate (equation 2).

Remember that hypoxia should normally drive a respiratory alkalosis (except in 'blue bloaters'). Think of pulmonary oedema and lung fibrosis – both may be associated with unremarkable chest X-rays. Inappropriately increased respiratory drive (amphetamines, panic attack, early salicylate poisoning).

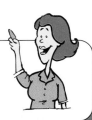

Q18

A 16-year-old boy has been receiving chemotherapy for a teratoma. He presents to casualty 3 days after his latest course in a confused state with hyperventilation.

INVESTIGATIONS	RESULTS
Arterial blood Po_2 (or PaO_2)	17.5 kPa
Arterial blood Pco_2 (or $PaCO_2$)	2.9 kPa
Plasma bicarbonate	12 mmol/l
Plasma sodium	135 mmol/l
Plasma potassium	7.2 mmol/l
Plasma chlorine	98 mmol/l
Plasma urea	45 mmol/l
Plasma creatinine	280 μmol/l
Plasma glucose	3.8 mmol/l

a) **What is the patient's anion gap?**

b) **What is the most likely diagnosis?**

c) **What would be your most important step in his immediate management?**

Aha! The bl**dy anion gap! Always a pain.

Actually, however, it is not so difficult.

MIND THE GAP

To maintain electrical neutrality in the blood, the concentration of cations and anions in the blood must be equal. However, the concentrations of routinely measured cations (sodium and potassium) and routinely-measured anions (chloride and bicarbonate) never match; there are many anions that are not measured. This concentration of unmeasured anions is called the 'anion gap'. In other words:

$$([Na^+] + [K^+]) - ([HCO_3^-] + [Cl^-]) = \text{the anion gap}$$

The anion gap is normally 15–20 mmol/l.

Thus, the presence of excess unmeasured acids will soak up buffering bicarbonate ions and the anion gap will increase. Coming up is a list of these situations. Cover it up now, and write down your own list, then check it against the table opposite.

CAUSES OF METABOLIC ACIDOSIS WITH HIGH ANION GAP

CONDITION	CAUSES
Ketoacidosis	Diabetic ketoacidosis
Lactic acidosis	
Type A (tissue hypoxia)	Circulatory shock (sepsis, cardiogenic shock, left ventricular failure, bleeds, severe anaemia)
Type B (no tissue hypoxia)	Acute hepatic failure
	Renal failure (acute and chronic)
	Leukaemias
	Biguanides (metformin, phenformin)
Poisoning with acids	Salicylates
	Methanol and ethanol

If the bicarbonate loss is matched by loss of cations, then the anion gap will be normal. Thus, when you see an acidosis with normal anion gap, think of conditions where bicarbonate and sodium/potassium are lost together. Write yourself a checklist now of such causes, and then compare it with the following list.

CAUSES OF METABOLIC ACIDOSIS WITH NORMAL ANION GAP

- Renal tubular acidosis

- Severe diarrhoea (remember villous adenomata, where potassium can be lost in quantity!)

- Carbonic anhydrase inhibitors (cause potassium and bicarbonate loss)

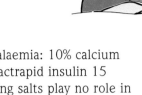

A18

a) Anion gap

32.2 mmol/l ($Na^+ + K^+ - Cl^- - HCO_3^-$)

b) Likely diagnosis

Tumour lysis syndrome

c) Immediate management

He needs emergency treatment of his hyperkalaemia: 10% calcium chloride 10 ml intravenous over 10 minutes, actrapid insulin 15 units, and 50% dextrose 50 ml. Calcium binding salts play no role in the acute management.

Here you are actually given the answer in the question. The patient is clearly in renal failure and you only have to make the obvious assumption that the cause of his renal failure is secondary to hyperuricaemia as a consequence of his chemotherapy. Such cases are quite rare these days, as patients are routinely predosed with allopurinol and preloaded with fluids. But that doesn't stop the examiners thinking that this is a good question.

LIVER LINE-UP

Fill in six causes of liver granulomata to reveal, in the grey boxes reading down, something to be big-headed about. See page 255 for the answers.

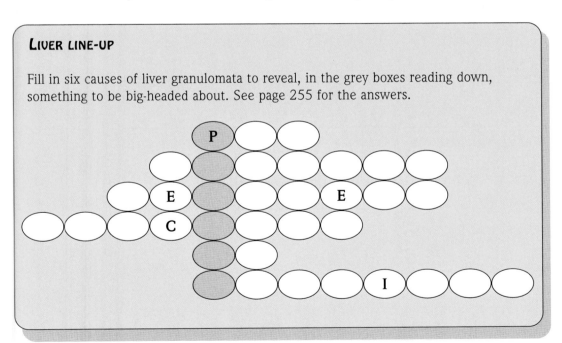

Q19 A 60-year-old woman presents to casualty with breathlessness. She has been increasingly short of breath over the last week. She is an ex-smoker of 10 pack years, but her husband continues to smoke 10–15 cigarettes per day. On direct questioning, she denies a cough productive of sputum, haemoptysis, or chest pain. She does voluntary work for her local church arranging flowers for weddings, and keeps a parrot. She returned from New Mexico 1 month ago, where she had been on holiday. She is diabetic and until recently was diet-controlled. However, she has recently put on 3 stone in weight ("but I hardly eat anything") and started oral hypoglycaemic agents 2 weeks ago.

ON EXAMINATION

- Body mass index = 32
- Respiratory rate = 34/min
- Early cataract in right eye

INVESTIGATIONS

- Haemoglobin = 12 g/dl
- Plasma sodium = 138 mmol/l
- Plasma glucose = 7.2 mmol/l
- White cell count = 7.1 x 10^9/l
- Plasma potassium = 4.6 mmol/l
- Plasma bicarbonate = 14 mmol/l
- Platelets = 382 x 10^9/l
- Plasma urea = 8.1 mmol/l
- Plasma chloride = 93 mmol/l
- Plasma creatinine = 112 μmol/l
- SaO_2 = 97%

SaO_2: oxygen saturation in arterial blood

a) What is the cause of her current presentation?

Hmmm. Not so straightforward at first glance. The history is full of red herrings, and most of the biochemistry, at first glance, looks pretty unremarkable. You know, by now, that there must be an abnormal finding with a limited list of causes. Either that, or this is a 'classic case' you just need to recognise.

Remember that breathlessness may be due to hypoxia, central drive abnormalities, or metabolic acidosis. Hypoxia is excluded by the normal SaO_2, and there is nothing to suggest a neurological component centrally. Thus, there is likely to be a metabolic acidosis.

Don't turn over for the answer, but calculate the anion gap.

The anion gap is high (35.6 mmol/l).

What are the causes of high anion gap metabolic acidosis? They are given earlier, but refresh your memory by filling in the table.

CONDITION	CAUSES
Ketoacidosis	
Lactic acidosis	
Type A (tissue hypoxia)	
Type B (no tissue hypoxia)	
Poisoning with acids	

We have no evidence of tissue hypoxia or ketoacidosis and she is unlikely to have been poisoned with methanol or salicylates.

Noninsulin dependent diabetes mellitus (NIDDM), overweight, new drug, thus suggests...

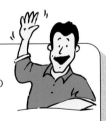

A19 a) **Cause of presentation**
Metformin, with compensatory hyperventilation due to metformin-induced lactic acidosis

Lessons to learn from this question

- If a new medication has recently been started, this is to be suspected as the cause or contributor to the pathology
- If the test results include chloride and bicarbonate, you're probably meant to use them!

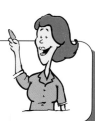

Q20

A 14-year-old girl presents to casualty with confusion. She is usually fit and well, apart from occasional headaches.

INVESTIGATIONS	RESULTS
Arterial blood pO_2 (or PaO_2)	17.3 kPa
Arterial blood pCO_2 (or $PaCO_2$)	2.2 kPa
Plasma bicarbonate	9 mmol/l
Plasma sodium	139 mmol/l
Plasma potassium	3.2 mmol/l
Plasma chloride	102 mmol/l
Plasma urea	6.3 mmol/l
Plasma creatinine	65 μmol/l
Plasma glucose	3.8 mmol/l

a) What investigation would you now order?

b) What is the most likely diagnosis?

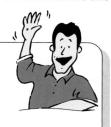

A20

a) Investigation
Salicylate levels

b) Likely diagnosis
Salicylate overdose

This is a severe metabolic acidosis with a high anion gap (31.2 mmol/l). The fact that she has intermittent headaches allows us to make the diagnosis of accidental salicylate overdose as being most likely. Salicylates may cause a primary respiratory alkalosis, a metabolic acidosis, tinnitus, deafness, visual obscurement, pulmonary oedema, renal failure, and hypoglycaemia.

A similar severe metabolic acidosis occurs in alcoholics who accidentally drink methanol. In the MRCP examination, the typical patient is a tramp, who is brought to casualty in a collapsed state from the local park, with a severe metabolic acidosis. In that case, the patient is meant to have drunk methylated spirits. Even if studies for the MRCP examination are not going well, we strongly advise you not to take this course of action. Like other activities said to be associated with solitary boredom, it can make you go blind.

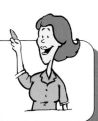

Q21

A 23-year-old woman presents to casualty on Christmas day with breathlessness. The casualty officer asks you to take a look at her blood gas results.

INVESTIGATIONS	RESULTS
Arterial blood pH	7.65
Arterial blood PaO_2	9.8 kPa
Arterial blood $PaCO_2$	7.8 kPa
Plasma bicarbonate	12 mmol/l
Base excess	−5
Plasma sodium	141 mmol/l
Plasma potassium	4.2 mmol/l
Plasma chloride	106 mmol/l
Plasma urea	3.3 mmol/l
Plasma glucose	4.1 mmol/l

a) What would you do next?

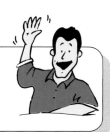

A21 a) **Action**
Repeat the blood gases and look at the patient!

This is a typical MRCP examination question that has come up on a number of occasions. Calculation shows she has a high anion gap (25.2 mmol/l). Furthermore, respiratory compensation for this would be to hyperventilate to blow off carbon dioxide, but this is also high. This suggests that she has a combined metabolic and respiratory acidosis, but in fact the pH shows she is alkalotic. Thus, the results are impossible and would need to be repeated. (A quick look at the patient should inform the experienced clinician that this is a load of nonsense.)

The clue in the question is that this occurred on Christmas day, and we can only conclude that either the casualty SHO or the laboratory technician overindulged in the Christmas spirit. But fortunately, you as the medical registrar will save the day. Hurrah!

Remember that, in the MRCP examination, trick questions such as this are loved by the examiners. They feel they are a good discriminator between candidates, although, with all the MRCP books and courses available, people fall for these less often.

Nonetheless, if a test does not appear to fit with the clinical situation then make sure that it is not a laboratory error.

Answers to Chorioidoretinitis causes (page 76): cytomegalovirus, syphilis, (boring), tuberculosis, toxocariasis, toxoplasmosis, (pimple), sarcoidosis.

Q22 A 63-year-old man who is otherwise fit and well presents to casualty 3 days after experiencing his first epileptic seizure. This occurred while he was working in his back garden and was witnessed by his wife who described a classic tonic–clonic grand mal seizure. At that time, he was seen by his GP who examined him and found no residual abnormality and arranged for an outpatient neurology referral. Since that time he has felt lethargic and slightly nauseous. He denies the consumption of excess alcohol or other drugs. It is noted in casualty that he is hyperventilating. The following are the results of his initial investigations.

INVESTIGATIONS	RESULTS
Arterial blood PaO_2	16.8 kPa
Arterial blood $PaCO_2$	3.8 kPa
Plasma bicarbonate	12 mmol/l
Arterial blood base excess	−7
Plasma sodium	141 mmol/l
Plasma potassium	4.2 mmol/l
Plasma chloride	106 mmol/l
Plasma urea	33.3 mmol/l
Plasma creatinine	290 μmol/l
Plasma glucose	4.1 mmol/l
Salicylates	Negative
CT head scan	NAD

NAD: no abnormality detected.

a) **What investigations would you make next?**

b) **What is the most likely diagnosis?**

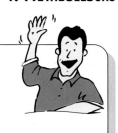

A22
a) **Investigations**
Urinary myoglobin, urinalysis, creatinine kinase
b) **Likely diagnosis**
Acute renal failure secondary to rhabdomyolysis

Again the clue to the question is the high anion gap metabolic acidosis. The cause of this is likely to be acute renal failure, and, given that he has had a grand mal seizure, the likely diagnosis is rhabdomyolysis as a consequence of this.

Rhabdomyolysis crops up in the MRCP examination on a regular basis. It can occur as a consequence of a number of medical problems (see below).

Causes of rhabdomyolysis

(TEASED)

Trauma – ischaemic muscle damage (compartment syndrome), bullet wounds, road traffic accidents

Exertion, if severe – paratroopers, prolonged epileptic seizures

Alcoholics – via seizures, prolonged immobility, hypophosphataemia

Snake bites!! (unusual, it has to said, in the UK)

Excessive temperature – malignant hyperthermia, or environmental

Drug intoxication – cocaine and Ecstasy, or prolonged immobility from any other cause

There is a range of congenital causes, but these are rare and seldom turn up in examinations. Feel free to look up McArdle's disease and mitochondrial diseases.

Treatment of rhabdomyolysis

- hydration – vigorous fluid replacement with central venous pressure measurements
- alkalinisation of the urine (keep urine pH > 7.6)
- dialysis if necessary

Useful information

One last problem that is unique to rhabdomyolysis-induced acute renal failure is the development of hypercalcaemia during the recovery phase in about one-third of patients. This complication can be prevented to some degree by avoiding calcium therapy of hyperkalaemia during the acute stage.

Q23

A young man is brought to casualty by his fiancée. She is worried that he is unable to walk without assistance. When he tries to demonstrate his gait, he is extremely unsteady and has a tendency to veer to one side. In addition to this, she has noticed that his speech has become more slurred in the last day or so. Initially she thought he had been drinking secretly, but his symptoms did not improve even after she poured all the alcohol away (except the Bailey's!). On examination, he is icteric with early clubbing of the nails. He is not pallid. He has 3 cm hepatomegaly and mild ascites. There is a resting tremor and he has an unsteady gait. He has no cerebellar signs or specific nerve palsies.

INVESTIGATION	RESULTS
Plasma sodium	140 mmol/l
Plasma bicarbonate	16 mmol/l
Plasma potassium	3.1 mmol/l
Plasma chloride	111 mmol/l
Plasma creatinine	102 μmol/l
Plasma glucose	5.6 mmol/l
Serum bilirubin	38 μmol/l
Serum alanine aminotransferase	80 IU/l
Serum alkaline phosphatase	130 IU/l
Arterial blood pH	7.29

a) What is the cause of this man's symptoms?

b) Can you explain the biochemistry results?

c) What is the underlying diagnosis?

d) What three investigations will confirm this?

e) What treatment should be started?

This man evidently has liver disease – presumably with portal hypertension producing the ascites. He also has some neurological signs. But what is the *key abnormal finding* for which there is *a limited list of diagnoses?*

As has been mentioned before, if bicarbonate and chloride levels are given, then use them! In this case, the anion gap is normal. You therefore need to go to the list of hypokalaemic acidosis with normal anion gap that was covered earlier.

Hypokalaemic acidosis with normal anion gap

'PARADE'

Partially-treated diabetic ketoacidosis (already acid: insulin drives potassium into cells)

Acetazolamide

Renal tubular Acidosis (type I = proximal, type II = distal)

Diarrhoea + hypovolaemic shock

Enteric (ureterosigmoidostomy or biliary/pancreatic fistula leading to bicarbonate loss: vipoma with MEN I)

MEN: multiple endocrine neoplasia.

Severe diarrhoea causes loss of sodium bicarbonate in stools followed by renal sodium chloride retention. Ureterosigmoidostomy causes chloride uptake in the bowel; this operation is becoming obsolete due to the fact that it causes a hyperchloraemic metabolic acidosis with increased blood ammonium and total-body potassium depletion. It is also associated with a 500-fold increase in the incidence of bowel cancer.

Biliary or pancreatic fistula

Vipoma with MEN I is also known as the Verner–Morrison syndrome.

By a process of elimination, we must be dealing with renal tubular acidosis. What are the causes of renal tubular acidosis, hepatocellular disease, and neurological signs? The answer is Wilson's disease.

You might approach this question in a number of ways. The 'list approach' narrows the diagnoses down, but eventually you need to 'just recognise the case'.

CAUSES OF RENAL TUBULAR ACIDOSIS	TYPE I	TYPE II
Idiopathic	–	–
Congenital	Autosomal dominant Autosomal recessive	Wilson's disease Cystinosis Galactosaemia Glycogen storage disease type I
Secondary	Rheumatoid arthritis Systemic lupus erythematosus Sjögren's syndrome Myeloma Cirrhosis Sickle cell anaemia	Heavy metals (cadmium, lead, and mercury) Amyloidosis PNH
Drug-induced	Ifosfamide Amphotericin Lithium	Carbonic anhydrase inhibitors Ifosfamide

PNH: paroxysmal nocturnal haemoglobinuria.

The heavy metal disorders are interesting and rare. Mercury is used in the treatment of vitiligo and homeopathic medicines, or accidentally leaked from power factories, so watch out! Cadmium toxicity causes osteomalacia with tubular changes and lung emphysema.

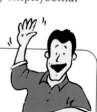

A23

a) **Symptom cause**
   Basal ganglia degeneration due to excess copper deposition

b) **Cause of biochemistry**
   Proximal (type II) renal tubular acidosis

c) **Diagnosis**
   Wilson's disease

d) **Investigations**
   Serum caeruloplasmin levels
   Urinary copper excretion
   Liver biopsy with rubianic acid staining

e) **Treatment**
   D-penicillamine to chelate excess circulating copper (modern treatment also requires zinc supplementation and molybdenum)

A common scenario...

...is to sling in a question where the urea is disproportionately raised compared to the creatinine (e.g. urea 38 mmol/l and creatinine 160 μmol/l). To work it out, just think of creatinine as coming from muscle.

Too much urea made   Huge high protein meal (and this includes a big upper GI bleed)

> Note: tetracycline prevents amino acid incorporation into protein. Amino acids are broken down to urea, raising the level inappropriately.

Low muscle mass   Old age with impaired renal function

    Bilateral amputee with impaired renal function

Dehydration is the commonest cause and steroid therapy is another (anabolism prevents muscle breakdown). Similarly, creatinine may be raised disproportionately in those receiving trimethoprim and cimetidine, as these drugs interfere with creatinine secretion and hence falsely raise levels in excess of the glomerular filtration rate. Liver failure and malnutrition will also reduce urea production.

As you may remember, this question comes up more often in the Part 1 MRCP examination, but has also appeared a number of times in Part II. Due to only a limited number of causes, this question is easy to answer.

Q24

A 21-year-old South African woman presented to casualty with a short history of abdominal pain and vomiting. She had been travelling around Europe with friends and had had no illnesses until now. Her current symptoms had started suddenly after a brief visit to Brighton, but she could not think of anything specific she could have eaten to cause this. She denied any diarrhoea or other symptoms.

On direct questioning she admitted to smoking occasionally, but denied illicit drug use and also claimed she did not drink alcohol, as it gave her a rash. Her only medication was the oral contraceptive pill, which she started recently.

ON EXAMINATION

- Temperature = 37.5°C
- Pulse = 110 beats/min regular
- Blood pressure = 170/110 mm/Hg
- Cardiovascular system = normal
- Respiratory system = normal
- Abdomen tender in epigastric region, bowel sounds active
- Marked blistering rash on face, hands, forearms, and shins

INVESTIGATIONS

- Haemoglobin = 13.5 g/dl
- Plasma sodium = 129 mmol/l
- Plasma potassium = 4.0 mmol/l
- Plasma urea = 8 mmol/l
- Plasma creatinine = 132 μmol/l
- WCC = 11 x 10⁹/l
- Neutrophils = 85%
- Platelets = 200 x 10⁹/l
- Amylase = normal
- Abdominal X-ray = NAD (remarkable)

NAD: no abnormality detected; WCC: white cell count.

a) **What is the diagnosis?**

b) **What one investigation would you do to confirm this?**

This is one of those questions where you either recognise the answer or you don't. It is not really a 'list' question. In fact, in real life, the cause of her abdominal pain could have been a dodgy curry (the infamous vindaloo revenge). But this is the MRCP examination!

The abnormal features are as follows:

- blistering photosensitive rash (distributed in 'exposed' areas)
- abdominal pain/tenderness
- tachycardia/hypertension/fever
- leucocytosis/SIADH
- rash with alcohol in a South African
- newly commenced oral contraceptive pill

A24

a) Diagnosis
The diagnosis to consider is variegate porphyria. This is not porphyria cutanea tarda, which is nonacute and doesn't cause abdominal pain, hypertension, or SIADH. Equally, this cannot be acute intermittent porphyria, as this is not associated with the photosensitive skin changes she reports. Having features of both clinches the diagnosis – if you knew this condition was more common in South Africans then you knew the answer before reading the whole question!

b) Investigation
Urinary protoporphyrinogen

BEFORE MOVING ON....

Quickly jot down the causes of:

• hyperparathyroidism

• bronchopulmonary eosinophilia

• lung cavitation

• hyponatraemia

- renal tubular acidosis

- angioid retinal streaks

- lung fibrosis

- hypokalaemic alkalosis and acidosis

FEATURES THAT SHOULD MAKE YOU THINK OF THE PORPHYRIAS

ACUTE PORPHYRIAS

Attacks are SADly (sulphonamides, alcohol, dieting) precipitated by the pill, pregnancy, 'phit' medicines (barbiturates, carbamazepine, phenytoin), and phevers (infection). There are two types: acute intermittent porphyria and variegate porphyria.

Acute intermittent porphyria (autosomal dominant)

GI:	Abdominal pain, vomiting, constipation
Neurological:	Peripheral, symmetrical motor neuropathy Occasional sensory symptoms/CNS palsies Epilepsy (20%) Papilloedema
Psychiatric:	Depression, hysteria, psychosis
General:	Fever, tachycardia, hypertension, leucocytosis, myocarditis and raised cholesterol
Investigations:	Elevated urea, abnormal liver function tests SIADH Elevated d-ALA (d-alanine) and porphobilogen (PBG) in urine Measure PBG-deaminase activity DNA screening
Treatment:	High carbohydrate diet, intravenous haematin (haem arginate), pain control with narcotic analgesics, β-blockers for hypertension, phenothiazines for psychological symptoms, anxiety, nausea, and vomiting, benzodiazepines and chloral hydrate for sedation and seizures; do not use conventional anticonvulsants (except gabapentin)

Variegate porphyria (autosomal dominant)

- South African
- neurological, abdominal, and general symptoms as above
- photosensitive blistering rash
- investigations: elevated urine protoporphyrinogen

NONACUTE PORPHYRIAS

Porphyria cutanea tarda (autosomal dominant or acquired)

Skin:	Fragility, photosensitive blistering rash Pruritus, milia, bullae, scars, hyperpigmentation Hirsutism
Metabolic:	Hepatomegaly, abnormal liver function tests Elevated serum iron and transferrin Diabetes
Investigations:	d-alanine and PBG are *never* elevated Elevated urinary uroporphyrin in attack Main precipitant is *alcohol*
Treatment:	Perform venesection (Hb <12 g/dl), give chloroquine and remove offending agents

Erythropoietic protoporphyria and congenital erythropoietic porphyria are other nonacute porphyrias.

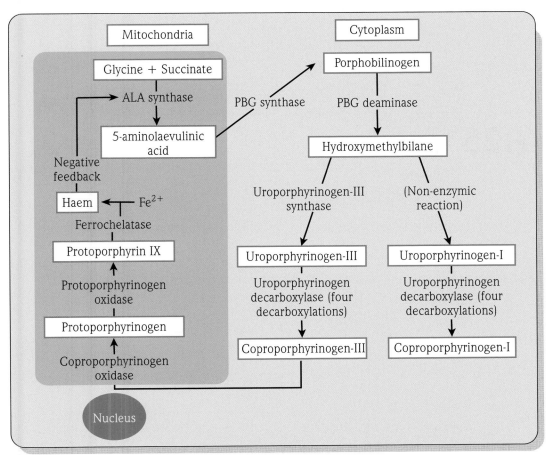

Q25

A 54-year-old man presents with glycosuria. He is a little overweight. His mother had NIDDM. He works as a fish-merchant and is an ex-petrol pump attendant. Two years ago he had a gastrectomy for a gastric carcinoma. He has been told he should have regular vitamin injections, but has been lax about this. He is otherwise well. He undergoes a glucose tolerance test.

• Time (hours)	0.0	0.5	1.0	1.5	2.0
• Serum glucose (mmol/l)	4.8	14.2	8.9	3.4	3.6

a) What is the result of the glucose tolerance test?

b) What is the likely cause in this man?

A25

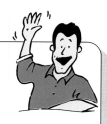

a) Test result
Lag storage curve

b) Likely cause
Post gastrectomy

Again this is just one of the classic glucose tolerance test results that are shown in the membership examination. The causes of a lag storage curve are:

- post gastrectomy
- liver failure

You have seen it now, so don't fall for it when it comes up in the data questions in the MRCP Part II.

5

HAVE A HEART...

THE CARDIOLOGICAL MRCP LISTS

There aren't really any long cardiology lists. Indeed, the variety of cardiological cases that seem to appear in the membership examination is quite small. Favourites are bacterial endocarditis and atrial myxoma: both can appear with symptoms of general malaise, weight loss, fever, arthralgia, haematuria, and strange symptoms due to emboli, which may be, for example, neurological, dermatological, or mesenteric. In addition, both conditions can produce a variety of autoantibodies at low titre. The differential diagnosis of such symptoms lies between these two conditions, autoimmune diseases such as polyarteritis nodosa and systemic lupus erythematosus (SLE), HIV, or tuberculosis (TB).

Causes of fever, haematuria, malaise, possible splenomegaly

- Polyarteritis nodosa
- SLE
- Bacterial endocarditis
- Left atrial myxoma
- Marantic endocarditis: found in those with malignancy, profound weight loss/cachexia
- Libman–Sacks endocarditis: an aseptic form of SLE endocarditis – previously thought to be benign, but can result in valve destruction and the need for surgery

The other pattern to recognise is that of cardiac failure and hepatomegaly. This is either due to hepatic engorgement from right heart failure, or an infection that 'attacks' both liver and heart, or to an infiltrative/deposition process affecting both organs. The choice is wide, but the 'likely lads' are listed below.

Causes of cardiac failure and hepatomegaly

- Congestive heart failure (with hepatic engorgement)
- Amyloidosis
- Lymphoma with cardiac involvement/tamponade
- Haemochromatosis
- Alcoholic cardiomyopathy
- Sarcoidosis

Q26

A 60-year-old Caucasian man presents to his local casualty department with an episode of haemoptysis. On further questioning he admits to being a heavy smoker, particularly since his wife died 18 months ago. He also admits that he has been feeling somewhat low and tired in the last 8 months. He thinks he may have lost some weight, but on direct questioning denies more specific symptoms other than more recently having a productive cough and increased sweating at night-time.

On examination

- Thin, cachectic with gingivitis
- Temperature = 38.5°C
- Pulse = 90 beats/min
- Blood pressure = 145/80 mmHg

Cardiovascular
- V waves visible in the JVP
- Heart sounds normal with a PSM audible at the left sternal edge, louder on inspiration

Respiratory
- Coarse crepitations throughout both lung fields

Abdomen
- No tenderness/organomegaly
- Normal rectal examination

Investigations

- Haemoglobin = 9.8 g/dl
- U&E = within normal limits
- WCC = 15.3 x 10^9/l
- Platelets = 431 x 10^9/l

Chest X-ray
- Increased cardiothoracic ratio
- Multiple rounded opacities in both lung fields

V: ventricular; JVP: jugulo-venous pressure; PSM: pansystolic murmur; U&E: urinalysis and electrolytes; WCC: white cell count.

a) **What is the most likely diagnosis?**

b) **What two investigations would be most helpful?**

This type of question can be difficult, as again there is so much 'social waffle'. Focusing on the purely pathological features should help sort out the wood from the trees.

The 'always pathological' list is:

- cachexia
- fever
- tricuspid regurgitation
- bilateral multiple rounded opacities on chest X-ray

Of course, cachexia and fever are pretty nonspecific. Immediate thoughts are usually of cancer or infection – or even both. Lung tumours often present with chest infection in the affected territory due to bronchial obstruction. We are not much further forward. However, tricuspid regurgitation does have a limited list of causes, and so do rounded lung opacities.

Write out the list of causes of multiple rounded lung opacities now. You should remember them from the 'Pants' section. If not, revise pages 61–62.

Tricuspid regurgitation

Tricuspid incompetence may be due to primary problems with the valve, or may be secondary to right heart dilatation or pressure overload.

Valve problems
- rheumatic heart disease
- bacterial endocarditis
- congenital heart disease (Ebstein's anomaly)
- carcinoid syndrome/slimming tablets
- myxomatous change

Secondary to elevated pulmonary artery pressures
- mitral valve disease
- cor pulmonale
- primary pulmonary hypertension

Secondary to right ventricular dilatation
- right ventricular infarction
- any dilated cardiomyopathy

Some of these conditions can immediately be discarded, as there is nothing to suggest them in either the history or examination. Put a line through these now. It then remains to select the cause that could most reasonably be expected to produce the chest X-ray appearance. As there is nothing in the history or examination to suggest a primary malignancy, and the patient has not complained of altered bowel habit, and has no hepatomegaly or flushing, it is unlikely that either pulmonary metastatic disease or carcinoid syndrome is the diagnosis.

This ought to leave you with one likely diagnosis. Check it by cross-indexing your list of causes of tricuspid regurgitation with the causes of *multiple well-rounded large opacities*:

- sarcoidosis
- metastases
- hydatid cysts
- abscesses
- septic emboli

Right-sided bacterial endocarditis seems to be the cause. Septic emboli have showered gradually to both lungs, initially causing few symptoms, but progressing of late. Although right-sided bacterial endocarditis is classically associated with intravenous drug abuse, it can also be associated with general debility. The examiners have given a clue – gingivitis as a source of infection.

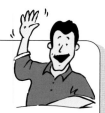

A26
a) **Diagnosis**
   Right-sided bacterial endocarditis with mycotic pulmonary emboli

b) **Investigations**
   Serial blood cultures
   Echocardiography with colour flow Doppler

EXTRA BITS: DOMINANT R-WAVES IN V1

Examiners always love electrocardiograms (ECGs) with a dominant R-wave in the right-side chest leads. This may be caused by:

- posterior myocardial infarction
- pulmonary embolus
- right ventricular hypertrophy (pulmonary hypertension/cor pulmonale/pulmonary stenosis, Noonan's syndrome and Duchenne's muscular dystrophy)
- right bundle branch block
- Wolff–Parkinson–White syndrome type A
- dextrocardia

Q27

A 45-year-old woman presents with a 3-week history of lethargy, malaise, and fever. One week before feeling unwell she had returned from a business trip in the Far East, but claims she had received all the requisite immunisations beforehand and whilst there only drank bottled water. Two weeks ago she began having intermittent left-sided abdominal pain and also noticed that her urine seemed pink. For the last 5 days she has had severe night sweats.

She presents today in a panic because she was transiently blind in her left eye for 2 hours this morning.

On examination

- No rash, lymphadenopathy or clubbing
- Temperature = 39°C
- Pulse = 110 beats/min regular
- Blood pressure = 145/60 mmHg

Cardiology
- Apex beat undisplaced
- Heart sounds normal, with pansystolic murmur heard at the apex
- Peripheral pulses all present and normal, with no bruits

Respiratory system
- Clear bilaterally

Neurology
- Normal central and peripheral nervous systems
- One small conjunctival haemorrhage noted

Abdomen
- Moderate tender splenomegaly
- No other organomegaly

Investigations

- Haemoglobin = 9.8 g/dl
- Plasma sodium = 140 mmol/l
- Plasma potassium = 6.1 mmol/l
- Urinalysis: blood + + +, protein +
- White cell count = 12.2 x 10^9/l
- Neutrophils = 90%
- Platelets = 500 x 10^9/l
- Erythrocyte sedimentation rate = 65 mm in first hour
- Rheumatoid factor positive at low titre
- Plasma urea = 45 mmol/l
- Plasma creatinine = 1035 μmol/l

Ultrasound abdomen
- Splenic enlargement with several high-density peripheral wedge-shaped areas
- Kidneys normal size

---

a) **What are the two main differential diagnoses to be considered?**

b) **What two investigations would be most helpful?**

The abnormal findings are:

- fever
- mitral incompetent murmur
- splenomegaly with evidence of splenic infarction
- conjunctival haemorrhage
- renal failure

In essence, this is a woman who has systemic symptoms (lethargy, malaise, fever, night sweats) and evidence of infection (raised white cell count, fever, raised platelet count and erythrocyte sedimentation rate [ESR]) accompanied by pathology of likely embolic origin, particularly transient blindness. We might also explain splenic infarction and conjunctival haemorrhage as being of embolic origin and renal failure as due to infection. The degree of renal failure might also suggest the development of rapidly progressive glomerulonephritis of which bacterial endocarditis is one of the causes. However, without an echocardiogram it would be difficult to favour one of these diagnoses over the other, as a significant number of renal embolic lesions may produce a similar degree of failure.

A weak positive rheumatoid factor is common in subacute bacterial endocarditis (SBE). So too are many other autoantibody tests (including P-ANCA [P-antineutrophil cytoplasmic antibody]). SBE is also a cause of decreased complement levels.

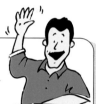

A27

a) **Differential diagnoses**
Left-sided bacterial endocarditis involving mitral valve, with systemic mycotic emboli
Left atrial myxoma with systemic embolisation

b) **Investigations**
Transoesophageal echocardiography
Serial blood and urine cultures

Q28

A 60-year-old woman is admitted as an emergency through casualty with severe breathlessness. This has progressed steadily over the last 3 months, initially with exertional shortness of breath, but now with paroxysmal nocturnal dyspnoea, orthopnoea requiring four pillows, and breathlessness at rest. Over the last 10 days, she has also noticed progressive swelling of her legs and intermittent abdominal pains.

She has had rheumatoid arthritis for the last 15 years. Currently this is quiescent, though she has required methotrexate and other disease-modifying medications in the past, and 4 months ago she was hospitalised for acute pain management and a course of penicillamine. She currently takes low-dose prednisolone together with nonsteroidal anti-inflammatory drugs (NSAIDs) as required. She has had asthma all her life, but tends to use her salbutamol inhaler only when it is cold. Otherwise she has no other illnesses and has never before been hospitalised. She recently retired, having spent the last 25 years working in human resources. She has just moved into a newly built house (which she has been redecorating), and lives with her husband of 45 years. On direct questioning she says she keeps two budgerigars and a pet vole.

ON EXAMINATION

- No cyanosis, lymphadenopathy, or clubbing
- Afebrile
- Pulse = 92 beats/min regular
- Blood pressure = 140/90 mm Hg

Cardiovascular
- JVP elevated 8 cm with positive Kussmaul's sign
- Apex beat 6th intercostal space, anterior axillary line
- Heart sounds: S1, S2+S3 gallop+S4
- Gross pitting oedema to mid-thigh

Respiratory
- Dull percussion note bibasally
- Reduced breath sounds bibasally, with inspiratory crepitations to mid-zone

Abdomen
- Abdomen soft, bowel sounds active, smooth hepatomegaly 4 cm, mild ascites

INVESTIGATIONS

- Full blood count = normal
- Plasma sodium = 134 mmol/l
- Plasma potassium = 3.8 mmol/l
- Serum albumin = 23 g/l
- Bilirubin = 17 μmol/l
- Plasma urea = 8 mmol/l
- Plasma creatinine = 175 mmol/l
- Serum alanine aminotransferase = 20 IU/l
- Serum alkaline phosphatase = 125 IU/l

Urinalysis
- Protein +++
- Blood trace
- 24-hour urine collection: 7 g/24 hour protein loss

ECG
- Right bundle branch block

Chest X-ray
- Bilateral upper lobe blood diversion
- Bilateral pleural effusions
- Alveolar shadowing

JVP: jugulo-venous pressure; ECG: electrocardiogram.

a) What is the most likely diagnosis?

_____

_____

b) How would you confirm this?

_____

Evidently, the patient has hepatomegaly and biventricular failure. You have already learned the causes for these. Write them down, then check them against the list on the next page.

_____

_____

_____

_____

_____

_____

_____

_____

_____

_____

_____

_____

_____

_____

_____

_____

_____

_____

_____

_____

Hepatomegaly with cardiac failure

- Congestive heart failure (due to valvular/cardiomyopathic/pericardial tamponade) with hepatic engorgement
- Amyloidosis
- Lymphoma with cardiac involvement/tamponade
- Haemochromatosis
- Alcoholic cardiomyopathy

Which of these is the likely cause? In this instance, the cardiac failure is due to a disease causing a restrictive cardiomyopathy or tamponade (Kussmaul's sign is positive). Which of these can cause nephrotic syndrome? You will find this list later in the book. In the meantime, your general knowledge ought to tell you.

A28

a) Diagnosis

You ought to be left with a differential diagnosis lying between Amyloidosis A, amyloidosis secondary to chronic rheumatoid arthritis, and haemochromatosis. In the absence of any features in the history pointing to haemochromatosis, amyloidosis must be the answer.

b) Investigation

The diagnosis is made by serum amyloid precursor (SAP) scanning or, better, organ biopsy of liver, right ventricle, or rectal tissue. A SAP scan uses a ^{123}I-isotope labelled amyloid precursor, which is injected and localises to areas of amyloid accumulation.

MORE QT, VICAR?

A long QT interval is a marker of abnormal ventricular repolarisation and is defined as a QTc (corrected for heart rate) greater than 450 ms. Pathological U waves may be present. Its most significant consequence is a predisposition to Torsades de Pointes.

CAUSES OF A LONG QT SYNDROME

Inherited long QT	Jervell and Lange–Nielsen syndrome and Romano–Ward syndrome
Electrolytes	Hypokalaemia, hypomagnesaemia, and hypocalcaemia
Endocrine disorders	Hypothyroidism, hyperparathyroidism, and phaeochromocytoma
Cardiac conditions	Chronic myocardial ischaemia, myocardial infarction, myocarditis, bradyarrhythmia, and atrioventricular (AV) node block
Intracranial disorders	SAH, encephalitis, and head trauma
Nutritional disorders	Anorexia nervosa and starvation
Drugs	Antiarrhythmic drugs: class IA/C, class III
	H1-receptor antagonists: terfenadine (no longer sold, do not combine with grapefruit juice)
	Cholinergic antagonists: cisapride, organophosphates
	Antibiotics: erythromycin, clarithromycin, trimethoprim
	Antifungal agents: ketoconazole, itraconazole
	Psychotropic agents: haloperidol, phenothiazines, and thioridazine
	Tricyclic antidepressants (especially in overdosage)

SAH: subarachnoid haemorrhage.

In Jervell and Lange–Nielsen syndrome (autosomal recessive, with sensorineural deafness) and Romano–Ward syndrome (autosomal dominant), mutations are in cardiac voltage-dependent sodium/potassium channel genes: *minK*, *MiRP1*, and *KVLQT1*. Patients tend to get arrhythmias if they are startled, for example, by the telephone ringing or other loud noises. They should be treated with prophylactic β-blockers. In acquired causes, give magnesium and avoid β-blockers, as these slow the heart and repolarisation. To speed the heart up and hence accelerate repolarisation, patients require pacing or catecholamine treatment.

If a patient presents with anything that might suggest an overdose, remember that tricyclic antidepressants are potent anticholinergic agents. In addition to causing tachycardias and arrhythmias, they cause a dry mouth, urinary retention, dilated pupils, and a lack of perspiration. Seizures, respiratory depression, and coma can occur. Always remember that depressed patients may also be taking other medications, such as lithium. Treatment of intractable arrhythmia in this context requires phenytoin. In examinations, beware of the patient with an overdose who has, for example, urinary retention (due to anticholinergic action from tricyclic antidepressants) and diabetes insipidus (lithium: renal toxicity).

6

SKINNY DIPS

DERMATOLOGICAL MRCP LISTS

Q29 A 27-year-old Afro-Caribbean woman presents with soreness on the anterior part of her shin. A palpable red lesion also appeared over the area concerned. She uses a salbutamol inhaler for asthma. Three years ago she had facial palsy, which resolved spontaneously. More recently, she gave birth to her second child and has begun treatment with oral contraceptives. A chest X-ray is reported as normal. The following investigations are performed.

INVESTIGATIONS	RESULTS
Full blood count	Normal
Urinalysis and electrolytes	Normal
Liver function tests	Normal
Serum calcium	2.75 mmol/l
Serum albumin	40 g/l
Serum phosphate	Normal
Parathyroid hormone	Normal
ACE	Normal
ASO titre	Negative
Mantoux test	Negative

ACE: angiotensin converting enzyme; ASO: antistreptolysin O.

a) What is the likely dermatological diagnosis for her shin lesion?

b) What is the most likely underlying diagnosis?

c) From her history is there another possible cause for her skin lesion?

This first part of this question is clearly easy, as the question gives you the clinical description of erythema nodosum. The difficult part is elucidating its cause. The patient has *hypercalcaemia.* Thus, the causes of erythema nodosum and hypercalcaemia need to be considered. Write down the causes of hypercalcaemia and then compare it to the list below.

Causes of erythema nodosum
- Sarcoidosis
- Tuberculosis (TB)
- Leprosy
- Inflammatory bowel disease
- Infections: streptococcal (β-haemolytic group A streptococci), histoplasmosis, coccidioidomycosis, and North American blastomycosis
- Drugs: oral contraceptive pills, sulphonamides, penicillins, bromides, and iodides

Or, put another (rather lavatorial) way, think of the stopcock: STOPCOCCiii
- Sarcoidosis
- TB
- Oral contraceptives
- Pills (sulphonamides, bromides, and iodides)
- StreptoCOCCi
- Inflammatory bowel disease
- Infections: histoplasmosis/coccidioidomycosis/blastomycosis

Or think of your own way of remembering it, and write it in the box below.

Erythema nodosum

The only conditions that appear in both lists are sarcoidosis and TB. Given that her chest X-ray is normal and that her Mantoux test is negative, this makes sarcoidosis the strongest possibility. A classic feature of sarcoidosis is anergy, which explains this test result. Furthermore, she has had facial palsy in the past, again suggesting the diagnosis of sarcoidosis.

The only problem now is to find another possible cause. Again the answer is in the question and this would suggest that the oral contraceptive pill is responsible.

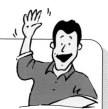

A29
a) **Dermatological diagnosis**
   Erythema nodosum

b) **Underlying diagnosis**
   Sarcoidosis

c) **Other possible cause**
   Oral contraceptive pill

QUIZ SPOT!

Q: Can you complete the rhyme about cavitating lesions in the lung?

_____ cause cavities, so can _____

_____, _____, also PE

Think of the 'oses' of which there are three

Also of abscesses, _____

A: See page 61 for the full rhyme.

Q30

A 23-year-old man is admitted to the casualty department with a 3-week history of shortness of breath. This has been associated with a fever and a cough productive of green-yellow sputum. He has a past medical history of asthma and hay fever. He is a smoker of 30 cigarettes per day and drinks 3 pints of lager per day.

On examination he is flushed, febrile at 38.2°C, with a rash on his back. The rash consists of multiple red circular lesions with a dusky centre. He has tachycardia with a pulse of 120 beats/minute. Chest expansion is reduced with bilateral basal inspiratory and expiratory coarse crackles.

INVESTIGATIONS	RESULTS
Haemoglobin	14.6 g/dl
White cell count	6.3 x 10^9/l
Platelets	324 x 10^9/l
Plasma sodium	134 mmol/l
Plasma potassium	4.2 mmol/l
Plasma creatinine	89 μmol/l
Plasma urea	4.3 mmol/l
Serum aspartate aminotransferase	34 (5–15) IU/l
Serum alanine aminotransferase	54 (5–15) IU/l
γ-glutamyl transferase	Normal
Serum alkaline phosphatase	Normal
HIV	Negative
Electrocardiogram	Normal
Chest X-ray	Bilateral basal consolidation
Blood cultures	Negative
ASO titre	Normal
Echocardiogram	Normal
Autoantibodies	Negative

ASO: antistreptolysin O. Figures in parentheses indicate normal ranges.

a) **What is the most likely diagnosis?**

b) **What two tests would you do to confirm the diagnosis?**

Again this is an easy question that we are sure you can get right by now!! (Well maybe.) This requires you to know the classic dermatological description of erythema multiforme and then correlate this with the clinical case scenario of a young man with progressive pneumonia and mild abnormalities of liver function.

CAUSES OF ERYTHEMA MULTIFORME

- Infections: herpes simplex virus (HSV) types I and II, Epstein–Barr virus (EBV), varicella zoster virus (VZV), adenovirus, hepatitis B/C viruses, *Mycoplasma*, *Streptococcus*, fungi
- Drugs: sulphonamides, sulphonylureas, nonsteroidal anti-inflammatory drugs (NSAIDs), anticonvulsants, and barbiturates
- Collagen vascular disease: systemic lupus erythematosus
- Malignancy: especially adenocarcinoma
- Sarcoidosis

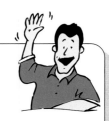

A30 a) **Diagnosis**
   Mycoplasma pneumoniae

b) **Investigations**
   Cold agglutinins, *Mycoplasma* serology

Note: The white cell count is often not raised with atypical pneumonias. Cold agglutinins are a feature of *Mycoplasma* infection. Other features of *M. pneumoniae* infection include sinusitis and haemorrhagic bullous myringitis, anaemia, low platelet count, hepatitis, pancreatitis, myocarditis, encephalitis, and cranial nerve palsies/Guillain–Barré syndrome.

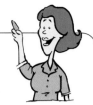

Q31

A 42-year-old man presents to casualty with a severe pain in the mouth and lips. He first noticed problems 2 days ago when he developed a number of skin lesions on his body and trunk. Over the next few days these coalesced and the skin around his mouth began to peel off. He is known to suffer from HIV infection and has had a previous episode of *Pneumocystis carinii* pneumonia (PCP) 2 years ago, since when he has received chemoprophylaxis. Currently his HIV is well controlled with a CD4 (T-helper cell) count of 390 cells/mm³, and an undetectable viral load with Combivir (zidovudine plus lamivudine) and nevirapine treatment.

On examination he is unwell and dehydrated with a temperature of 38.5°C. The skin around his mouth is denuded, as is the skin on his tongue. Over his body there are multiple coalescing erythematous target lesions. Chest examination is unremarkable and his abdomen is soft and nontender.

INVESTIGATIONS	RESULTS
Haemoglobin	12.6 g/dl
Mean corpuscular volume	100 fl
White cell count	6.9 x 10⁹/l
Platelets	360 x 10⁹/l
Urinalysis and electrolytes	Normal
Liver function tests	Normal
ASO titre	Negative
Chest X-ray	Normal

ASO: antistreptolysin O.

a) What is the most likely diagnosis?

b) What two things would you do next?

Again the history gives a classic description of erythema multiforme, but this time it is complicated by the fact that the patient is HIV positive. This therefore requires a further list of complications of HIV therapy, and we need to cross-reference this with the list of causes of erythema multiforme. Write down the possible causes of erythema multiforme and compare it to the table below.

NUCLEOSIDE ANALOGUES	NON-NUCLEOSIDE ANALOGUES	PROTEASE INHIBITORS
Azidothymidine/ zidovudine (AZT): • macrocytosis • pancytopenia • black nails Dideoxycytidine (DDC)/ dideoxyinosine (DDI): • pancreatitis Lamivudine: • nausea and vomiting Stavudine: • peripheral neuropathy	Efavirenz: • nightmares • skin rash Nevirapine: • skin rashes, including erythema multiforme and Stevens–Johnson syndrome	Indinavir: • renal stones • vomiting and diarrhoea • mitochondrial toxicity* • lipodystrophy** Ritonavir: • vomiting and diarrhoea • mitochondrial toxicity* • lipodystrophy

*   Mitochondrial toxicity presents with lactic acidosis and fatty liver.

** Lipodystrophy presents with: high cholesterol and triglycerides, diabetes, fat redistribution including a buffalo hump, abdominal distension, and facial lipodystrophy.

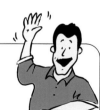

A31

a) Likely diagnosis
Stevens–Johnson syndrome caused by either co-trimoxazole (as prophylaxis against PCP) or nevirapine

b) Management
Withdraw the offending drug, rehydrate, give steroid therapy (however, none of these are thought to be helpful in nevirapine-induced Stevens–Johnson syndrome)

Q32 A 21-year-old man presents to casualty with a large necrotic ulcer on his right shin that first appeared 3 weeks earlier. On examination, he is a thin man with digital clubbing and a colostomy. He has previously suffered from mild epilepsy and hypertension. He is not currently on any medication for these conditions. He has an elder brother who has asthma.

a) What is the most likely cause of his skin condition?

b) Why has he got a colostomy?

Again this question is easy, as long as you know the causes of pyoderma gangrenosum and clubbing. These are recorded for you below.

CAUSES OF PYODERMA GANGRENOSUM

- Inflammatory bowel disease
- Myeloma
- Acute myeloblastic leukaemia (AML)
- Polycythaemia rubra vera
- IgA paraproteinaemia
- Connective tissue diseases: systemic lupus erythematosus, rheumatoid arthritis, polyarteritis nodosa

CAUSES OF CLUBBING

- Congenital
- Cardiac: sub-acute bacterial endocarditis
                 atrial myxoma
                 congenital cyanotic heart disease
- Respiratory: carcinoma of bronchus
                 bronchiectasis
                 cystic fibrosis
                 pulmonary fibrosis
                 mesothelioma
- GI: inflammatory bowel disease
                 liver cirrhosis
                 coeliac disease
- Endocrine: thyroid acropachy

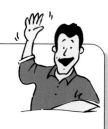

A32   **a) Likely cause of skin condition**
          Pyoderma gangrenosum

          b) Cause of colostomy
          Ulcerative colitis

Use the space below to come up with ways of remembering these lists. You could use mnemonics, verse, pictures, alliteration (same letters), or biological classifications.

Quiz Spot!

Presentation Puzzle

George, Michael, Sarah, Nicky, Peter and Ruth are six members of the Job family and all suffer from four presenting conditions, A–D. Some are unlucky in that they have contracted large numbers of diseases. Others are unlucky in that a single disease has led to more than one clinical presentation. Which disease states are responsible for each finding in each patient? Write one causal disease in each box. The answers are on page 234, but the following information may help:

1. Michael has one disease responsible for more than two of his clinical presentations.
2. Sarcoid causes George's bilateral hilar lymphadenopathy, and also his lung fibrosis.
3. Sarah has recent abdominal swelling and a positive B-HCG.
4. Michael and Nicky share an infective cause of thenar eminence wasting.
5. Michael and Sarah share a cause of chronic sputum production.
6. Ruth does not have any infectious diseases.
7. One man has cystic fibrosis as a cause of two conditions.
8. The person with an autoimmune joint disease also has yellow nails.
9. The girl who keeps pigeons is also pregnant.
10. Sarah gave Nicky an infectious disease.
11. The girl who gave the infectious disease to Michael also has a fungal infection.
12. The man with cystic fibrosis has a GP who thinks that amiodarone is a treatment for gout.
13. The acromegalic has Kartagener's syndrome.
14. The girl with extrinsic allergic alveolitis also has rheumatoid arthritis.

	Presenting condition			
	A	B	C	D
George				
Michael				
Sarah				
Nicky				
Peter				
Ruth				

Which two are the least infected?
In which patients may serum ACE be elevated?

7

GASTROINTESTINAL TRACTS

THE GI MRCP LISTS

Q33 There are several list structures that you should know by heart by now. For instance, the causes of ascites may be divided by the nature of the ascitic tap: transudates which are due to low plasma oncotic pressure or high capillary pressure, exudates which can be inflammatory, and chylous (lymph fluid). Complete your own table of causes below.

CHYLOUS										

EXUDATES										

TRANSUDATES	High capillary pressure									
	Low oncotic pressure									

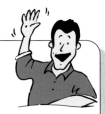

A33

TRANSUDATES

can be caused by a low plasma protein due to not eating enough (such as kwashiorkor), not synthesising enough (all causes of liver failure), or to losing protein. Remember that you can lose protein from the kidneys (nephrotic syndrome) and gut (protein losing enteropathy, which may complicate any inflammation of the bowel). Or you can have high capillary pressure of cardiac origin (remember all causes of right heart failure and constrictive pericarditis) or of local origin (remember compression of the portal vein by tumour or portal nodes, as well as destruction of the liver architecture in cirrhosis).

EXUDATES

Meanwhile, any local infection or inflammation will produce an exudate. In particular, remember Budd–Chiari syndrome and tuberculosis (TB) as causes.

JAUNDICE

Jaundice is also a common enough clinical finding, and the causes (as you also ought to know well) may be divided into pre-hepatic (or haemolytic), hepatic (or hepatocellular), and post-hepatic (or obstructive). You ought to be able to come up with your own list of causes for each of these. Jot them down now to remind yourself.

There are, however, one or two classic causes that might need a little neuronal refreshment. These are Gilbert's syndrome, Crigler–Najjar syndrome, Dubin–Johnson syndrome, and Rotor's syndrome. Remember that the 'i's are the 'un's: Gilbert's syndrome, and Crigler–Najjar syndrome produce **un**conjugated hyperbilirubinaemia, and Rotor's and Dubin–Johnson syndromes produce conjugated. As Crigler–Najjar syndrome is usually fatal in the first year of life, in adults you only need to consider the other three.

BILIRUBIN	SYNDROME	INHERITANCE	COMMENTS
Unconjugated	Gilbert's	Autosomal dominant	UDPGT deficiency, SBR usually <35 μmol/l, fasting and intravenous nicotinic acid cause a rise in SBR, no haemolysis, normal LFTs, benign course
	Crigler–Najjar	Autosomal recessive	Similar to Gilbert's, but very rare and presents in neonates as kernicterus. Type I has no UDPGT, type II has some, which can be induced with phenobarbitone
Conjugated	Dubin–Johnson	Autosomal recessive	Conjugated bilirubin $+++$, black-pigmented liver biopsy, right upper quadrant pain, malaise, fatigue, and no gallbladder seen on oral cholecystogram
			Bromsulphthalein test shows early clearance at 45 min, and late rise at 90 min
	Rotor's	Autosomal recessive	No significant clinical jaundice, normal liver biopsy

LFTs: liver function tests; SBR: serum bilirubin; UDPGT: uridine diphosphateglucuronosyl transferase.

CATCH POINT

Always remember that, whatever the case in the MRCP, drugs may be responsible. Don't be caught out. "It's the tablets what's doin' it, doc" is very true as far as the examiners are concerned. For example, in a case of intermittent ataxia, consider whether the child might be eating granny's phenytoin.

Jaundice may also be due to drugs, either through haemolysis (virtually anything will cause this), hepatotoxicity, or intrahepatic cholestasis. Any drug can, in theory, cause jaundice. Thus, you should think of this as a cause, and there is little point in learning an exhaustive list. But just for fun...

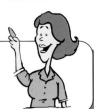

Q34 a) Name four drugs that may cause intrahepatic cholestasis

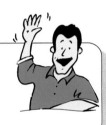

A34 a) **Drugs causing intrahepatic cholestasis**

Chlorpromazine, imipramine, sulphonamides, erythromycin estolate, nitrofurantoin, chlorpropamide ...and, yes, there are loads more too.

CLASSIC CASES

PERNICIOUS ANAEMIA

You will remember that pernicious anaemia is associated with lack of intrinsic factor and achlorhydria. Most (>90%) have antiparietal cell antibodies. Watch out, therefore, for pernicious anaemia in any case in which the mean corpuscular volume (MCV) is high, or when another autoimmune disease is present (30% of those with myxoedema have pernicious anaemia). Also watch out for the presence of other associated features:

- mild splenomegaly, mild haemolysis, a hypocellular bone marrow
- hypogammaglobulinaemia and IgA deficiency
- reticulocytosis with treatment
- achlorhydria
- the association with stomach cancer (4%)
- *Salmonella* osteomyelitis as a rare association

QUIZ SPOT!

CAUSES OF ERYTHEMA NODOSUM

Starting with the shaded square, move in any direction (single squares only, no diagonals) to find the causes of erythema nodosum. Just to muck things up, there is a sporting animal and a few beasts of burden in there too. What are they? See page 83 for the answers.

S	T	Y	C	I	S	D	E	O	D
A	O	M	O	S	M	I	S	I	I
L	I	P	T	B	O	R	B	E	D
B	L	E	H	T	S	I	S	S	S
S	L	S	U	S	A	S	E	R	T
I	M	S	L	C	R	O	D	E	M
S	O	A	P	O	I	D	I	P	U
S	T	L	H	O	N	A	M	T	L
I	O	P	H	O	R	S	S	O	E
H	D	B	I	I	C	C	O	C	S

BLOODY DIARRHOEA, AGAIN!!!

The presence of bloody diarrhoea can be the clue to grey cases, and is often mentioned "in passing" if you will excuse the pun. However, all causes are associated with systemic symptoms and complications that are often laboured.

All causes may lead to renal failure due to the septic state and to dehydration, and to haemolytic uraemic syndrome (HUS) in the case of *Escherichia coli*.

Salmonella typhi

Typhoid is faeco-orally transmitted, and may be associated with pancytopenia, osteomyelitis (in pernicious anaemia and sickle cell disease), and perforation (rarely). Typhoid presents with:

- week 1: fever, malaise, constipation, headache, dry cough, confusion, abdominal pain
- week 2 (hits Peyer's patches): diarrhoea, rose spots, splenomegaly, leucopenia and virtually any 'itis' (osteomyelitis, meningitis, myocarditis)
- week 3: gastrointestinal bleed, perforation

In week 1, 90% are blood culture positive. In week 2, bone marrow/stool/urine cultures are more likely to be positive. The analytical protein index (API) and Widal's reaction (serum agglutinins for the O and H antigens) can also be used for diagnosis.

Salmonella typhimurium (or Dublin)

S. typhimurium is a zoonosis. Watch out for sausages, curried eggs, frozen chicken curry, and Edwina Curry. Watch out, as it causes a septic state and ends up anywhere; hence meningitis, pyelonephritis, splenic abscess, skin lesions.

Shigella/E. coli

Note that verotoxin 0157-producing strains of *E. coli* may cause HUS.

Campylobacter

Campylobacter is caught from puppies, pecked milk-bottles, and chicken and is often associated with severe systemic symptoms, such as headache and severe myalgia.

Amoebiasis

Amoebiasis may 'rear' its head long (even years) after exposure, and may present with an abdominal mass, with or without obstruction, or abscess; always think of abscess in the presence of unexplained fever, malaise, and weight loss. Other causes to note are endocarditis, lymphoma, solid malignancies, polymyositis and vasculitis.

Diverticulitis

Diverticulitis may be a cause of bloody diarrhoea, and like any other sepsis may be associated with portal pyaemia and severe illness, as well as perforation, abscess (see above), fistula, and obstruction.

Ulcerative colitis and Crohn's disease

Both of these conditions may be associated with malignant conversion, seronegative arthritides, mouth ulcers, iritis, autoimmune hepatitis, cholangitis, and amyloidosis. Drug treatment may be the cause of a rash or pancytopenia.

Remember that terminal ileitis may be caused by Crohn's disease and tuberculosis (TB), the common differential, as well as *Yersinia*. It may also be mimicked by a tumour.

Ischaemic colitis

This should be considered in the presence of other vascular disease, or mesenteric angina. Sudden onset of bloody diarrhoea should make you think of embolisation of: clot (atrial fibrillation), immune complexes (subacute bacterial endocarditis), or tumour (atrial myxoma).

Carcinoma

This may present in a number of ways, which you should be aware of.

CAUSES OF CIRRHOSIS

•	Congenital:	Haemochromatosis and Wilson's disease
		α_1–antitrypsin (remember early emphysema)
		Galactosaemia
		Type IV glycogenosis
•	Infectious:	Chronic active hepatitis (hepatitis B and C)
•	Immunological:	Primary biliary cirrhosis and autoimmune hepatitis
•	Prolonged cholestasis:	Secondary biliary cirrhosis
•	Vascular diseases:	Congestive heart failure, hepatic vein thrombosis, Rendu–Osler–Weber syndrome
•	Adverse drug reactions:	Methotrexate, methyldopa, sulphonamides, isoniazid, carbon tetrachloride, amiodarone
•	Cryptogenic	

Malabsorption

This sneaks in under all sorts of guises, usually of the deficiency variety. This means the presence of oedema (protein deficiency), bleeding (vitamin K), neuropathies (vitamin B_{12} or folate deficiency), or anaemia (macrocytic due to vitamin B_{12} deficiency usually: iron deficiency due to malabsorption is unusual, and you should consider hookworm as a cause of a mixed deficiency picture). In addition, the case may be presented as a specific complication of one of the causes, such as one of the associated complications of Crohn's disease and ulcerative colitis (above) or of coeliac disease.

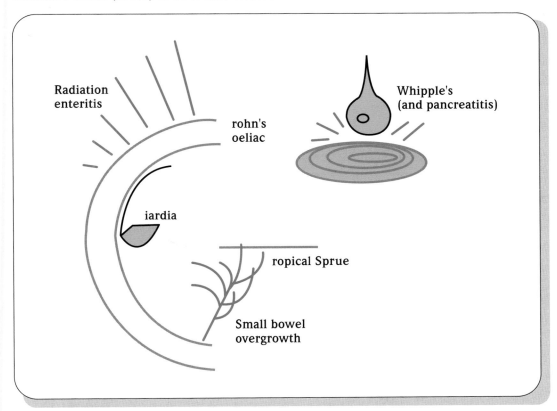

Causes of malabsorption

Most of these cause malabsorption through villous atrophy. Tropical sprue is a tropical form of post-enteritis villous atrophy, and is treated with tetracycline and folic acid. Coeliac disease is due to gluten insensitivity and may be associated with hyposplenism and dermatitis herpetiformis, which is characterised by symmetrical itchy urticaria on extensor aspects of the limbs, gluteal regions, and interscapular that becomes vesicular. Post-enteritis villous atrophy can occur after any infectious diarrhoea. Lymphoma of the small bowel is also a cause.

Q35

A 35-year-old health visitor presents to casualty with a 6-month history of lower abdominal pain, altered bowel habit with frequent diarrhoea, and weight loss of nearly 1 stone in the same period. She came to the UK at the age of 12 years with her parents and visited Pakistan once a year to see her grandparents until 4 years ago when they died within months of each other. She has suffered chronic constipation, strains at stool, and has recently been diagnosed as suffering from haemorrhoids. Her doctor says she 'needs vitamins'. She doesn't smoke or drink alcohol. Her husband is a regular attendee at the diabetic clinic.

ON EXAMINATION

- Thin, pale but not clubbed, cyanosed, or jaundiced
- Temperature = 37.5°C
- Pulse = 98 beats/min regular
- Blood pressure = 130/85 mmHg
- No lymphadenopathy
- Cardiovascular system = normal
- Respiratory system = normal
- Abdominal examination reveals a globally tender abdomen, with a mass in the right iliac fossa.
- Normal rectal examination

INVESTIGATIONS

- Haemoglobin = 9.5 g/dl
- Plasma sodium = 136 mmol/l
- Plasma potassium = 3.2 mmol/l
- White cell count = 13 x 10⁹/l
- Platelets = 450 x 10⁹/l
- Plasma urea = 4.5 mmol/l
- Serum albumin = 30 g/l
- Other liver function tests = normal
- ESR = 78 mm in first hour
- Stool microscopy: no ova, cysts, or parasites
- Chest X-ray: normal, clear lung fields, two calcified nodules in right hilum

ESR: erythrocyte sedimentation rate.

a) Give three possible diagnoses

b) Give three appropriate investigations to differentiate between these

This is one of those 'you get it or you don't' questions. This scenario (or one like it) is much loved by membership examiners (bless their little hearts). The patient has:

- systemic features (weight loss, anaemia, fever)

- right iliac fossa mass and nonbloody diarrhoea

- hilar calcified nodules

The 'not-very-well-with-mass-in-the-right-iliac-fossa' story has three possible conclusions: cancer (especially small bowel lymphoma), ileocaecal TB, or Crohn's disease. The Indian origin and nodules are meant, in this case, to suggest TB.

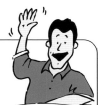

A35 **a) Possible diagnoses**
Ileocaecal tuberculosis
Terminal ileal Crohn's disease
Small bowel lymphoma
(Could also be *Yersinia* enterocolitis or actinomycosis)

b) Investigations
Colonoscopy and biopsy and culture
Small bowel meal and follow-through
Abdominal ultrasound

(Stool culture for TB gets fewer marks, as the test may be negative and takes a long time.)

TIP

There is a rule that disease of the terminal ileum affects vitamin B_{12}/folate absorption more than iron absorption. The reverse is true for disease that affects the duodenum (e.g. coeliac disease) and this may be useful in helping to distinguish different disease processes.

QUICK CHECK

Jot down the causes of:

- porphyria
- polycythaemia
- polyarthropathy
- optic atrophy

- high anion-gap acidosis
- lung cavitation
- erythema nodosum

Q36

A 55-year-old company director presents with a 4-month history of weight loss and abdominal pain. The pain is intermittent and is associated with what the patient describes as the passage of "putty coloured" stools. Despite this he has a good appetite and is surprised that he has lost almost 8 kg in weight. On direct questioning he admits to sweating more of late, but not possessing a thermometer he is unaware of whether he has had a fever. He travels often with his work, primarily to New York, Tokyo, and Lagos, but insists he has had all the requisite immunisations, and denies extra-marital liaisons or the use of illicit drugs. He smokes 10 cigarettes per day and restricts his alcohol intake to 1–2 whiskeys with clients. His only other medical problem is a 10-year history of recurrent painless swelling of his wrists, knees, and ankles, which seems to settle spontaneously. He has never sought medical advice regarding this.

ON EXAMINATION

- Very tanned but anaemic, with cervical and supraclavicular lymphadenopathy
- Temperature = 37.5°C
- Pulse and blood pressure = normal
- Early clubbing
- Joints normal
- Abdominal examination reveals diffuse tenderness, but no organomegaly or masses

INVESTIGATIONS

- Haemoglobin = 9.5 g/dl
- Plasma sodium = 138 mmol/l
- Plasma potassium = 3.3 mmol/l
- Plasma glucose = 5.3 mmol/l
- Plasma urea = 6.5 mmol/l
- Serum albumin = 25 g/l
- Plasma creatinine = 95 μmol/l
- White cell count = 7.5 x 10^9/l
- Platelets = 212 x 10^9/l
- ESR = 80 mm in first hour
- Mean corpuscular volume = 105 fl
- Serum ACE = 100 U/l
- Stool microscopy negative for ova, cysts, and parasites
- Jejunal biopsy shows jejunal villous atrophy
- CT abdomen shows para-aortic lymphadenopathy

ACE: angiotensin converting enzyme, CT: computed tomography; ESR: erythrocyte sedimentation rate.

a) **What is the diagnosis?**

_____

b) **How would you confirm this?**

_____

c) **What treatment would you give?**

_____

He has:

- systemic features (weight loss, fever, sweating)
- lymphadenopathy
- small bowel malabsorption secondary to jejunal villous atrophy (steatorrhoea, weight loss, macrocytic anaemia)
- large joint arthropathy (preceding the onset of gastrointestinal upset).

Remember Occam's razor and the principle of scientific parsimony and try to find _one_ unifying diagnosis, rather than making additional assumptions about the relevance of clearly pathological findings.

Start with a list you have already learned: the causes of polyarthropathy.

POLYARTHROPATHY

Joint attacks are done by three –

_____, _____, _and_ _____

_____, _____,

And _____

_____, _____, _____, _____,

_____, _____, _____

_Spread by_____ _(and not by_ _____ _)_

Is the dreaded _____

_____, _____, _____

_____

Coming over _____

With widespread _____

_____, _and_ _____ _do_

Chronic _____ too

_____ and _____, _never fear!_

_____ shall bring up 'the rear'!

WHICH OF THESE IS ASSOCIATED WITH BOWEL DISEASE?

Five patterns fit the bill:

- inflammatory bowel disease (IBD: ulcerative colitis or Crohn's disease) plus ankylosing spondylitis (not related to disease activity)
- IBD (ulcerative colitis or Crohn's disease) plus enteropathic synovitis (related to disease activity)
- autoimmune chronic active hepatitis (CAH) plus bilateral symmetrical small joint arthropathy
- Whipple's disease plus large joint arthropathy (often precedes gastrointestinal symptoms)
- familial Mediterranean fever (FMF) plus monoarticular arthritis

The diagnosis has been narrowed down to FMF, Whipple's disease, CAH, or IBD.

SMALL BOWEL MALABSORPTION

Earlier it was established that there are few causes of small bowel malabsorption. Most of the causes are through villous atrophy. Tropical sprue is a tropical form of post-enteritis villous atrophy, which can occur after any infectious diarrhoea and is treated with tetracycline and folic acid. Coeliac disease is due to gluten insensitivity and may be associated with hyposplenism and dermatitis herpetiformis (symmetrical itchy urticaria on extensor aspects of the limbs, gluteal regions, and interscapular that becomes vesicular). Lymphoma of the small bowel is also a cause.

Thus, the differential diagnosis of jejunal villous atrophy is:

- coeliac disease
- infectious enteritis
- gastrointestinal lymphoma
- Whipple's disease
- tropical sprue
- HIV

Thus, the only overlap on the lists for polyarthropathy, bowel disease, and jejunal villous atrophy is Whipple's disease. IBD, FMF, and CAH have been excluded.

A36

a) Diagnosis

Whipple's disease

b) Tests

Periodic acid-Schiff (PAS) staining of jejunal biopsy sample: the macrophages in the section stain strongly with PAS and contain the intracellular bacilli of *Tropheryma whippelii*. Alternatively, polymerase chain reaction may detect *T. whippelii* DNA on biopsy samples.

c) Treatment

Penicillin, tetracycline, co-trimoxazole, or chloramphenicol for 6–24 months with or without steroids

WHIPPLE'S DISEASE

Whipple's disease is a rare (except in the MRCP examination!) multi-system disorder that is more common in those who are HLA-B27 (human leucocyte antigen B27) positive. It most commonly affects the small bowel, but extra-intestinal features frequently precede the malabsorption. Other associated features of Whipple's disease include:

- joints: large joint arthropathy
- heart: endocardial, myocardial, pericardial involvement with heart failure
- lungs: pleural effusion, pulmonary oedema
- central nervous system: cranial nerve palsies, aseptic meningitis, ataxia, dementia
- skin: hyperpigmentation and photosensitivity
- other: splenomegaly, glossitis, and lymphadenopathy

Draw yourself a cartoon on the next page of a classic patient with Whipple's disease. Learn to draw it repeatedly, so that you remember the features.

Whipple's disease also shares several features with sarcoidosis, frequently leading to confusion. Such features include elevated serum ACE, the appearance of epithelioid granulomas on lymph node biopsy, and an occasional improvement with steroids.

Note that all causes of small bowel malabsorption may cause hyperpigmentation. (In this question, for 'tanned' read 'hyperpigmented'.) The 'hyperpigmented' list, therefore, includes: malabsorption, haemochromatosis, copper storage diseases, amiodarone treatment, Addison's disease, and Nelson's syndrome.

Your cartoon of a classic patient with Whipple's disease

Extra bits: autoimmune liver disease

Examiners will often try to catch you out by making the presenting complaints (or dominant pathological findings) due not to the liver disease itself, but to the sequelae of chronic liver disease. These include the 'medical student' list (e.g. gynaecomastia, liver flap, Dupuytren's contracture), but also HePatic COMAX:

- hyponatraemia
- peripheral neuropathy from vitamin deficiency
- coagulopathies
- osteomalacia from malabsorption
- malabsorptive diarrhoea
- ascites
- xanthelasmata

You have to be especially alert for the association of autoimmune liver disease with other autoimmune diseases, which may have a greater focus in the question. The two commonest autoimmune diseases to focus on for examinations are primary biliary cirrhosis and chronic active hepatitis.

PRIMARY BILIARY CIRRHOSIS

- Histologically: periportal fibrosis, Mallory bodies, and liver granulomata (see 'other causes of liver granulomata', below). The mention of copper deposition is meant to fool you into diagnosing Wilson's disease (in which Mallory bodies and granulomata are not seen)
- Associated with rheumatoid arthritis, CREST syndrome, Sjögren's syndrome, Hashimoto's disease, coeliac disease, dermatomyositis, and renal tubular acidosis
- Clinically may be associated with peptic ulcer and may be triggered by the pill or pregnancy
- Also associated with very high levels of alkaline phosphatase, gamma glutamyl transferase, cholesterol, and IgM antimitochondrial antibodies

CHRONIC ACTIVE HEPATITIS

- Histologically: macronodular cirrhosis, periportal inflammation, piecemeal necrosis (the latter is not seen in primary biliary cirrhosis)
- Associated with viral hepatitis (hepatitis B, particularly if e antigen is positive), Wilson's disease
- Associated with drug use, such as methyldopa or isoniazid
- Associated with autoimmunity (50% of cases of ulcerative colitis)

The presence of antismooth muscle, antinuclear, and antimitochondrial antibodies is common in both primary biliary cirrhosis and chronic active hepatitis. The presence of anticentromere antibodies suggests systemic sclerosis as a cause, where as speckled antinuclear antibody suggests mixed connective tissue disease.

OTHER CAUSES OF LIVER GRANULOMATA

- Classic granulomatous disease: sarcoidosis, TB, Wegener's granulomatosis, *Brucella*, berylliosis
- Other autoimmune disease: IBD, polyarteritis nodosa, giant cell arteritis
- Infections (T²AG along and C⁴): tropical (leprosy, schistosomiasis), toxocariasis, ascariasis, giardiasis, and *Coxiella*, Cytomegalovirus, coccidiodomycosis, clap (syphilis)
- Malignancies, drugs, and the chronic granulomatous diseases

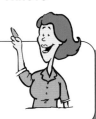

Q37

A 15-year-old girl presents to the clinic with weight gain and nausea for the last 2 months. A number of investigations are ordered.

Investigations	Results
Haemoglobin	11.1 x 10⁹/l
White cell count	3.8 x 10⁹/l
Platelets	234 x 10⁹/l
Plasma calcium	Normal
Serum bilirubin	6 (3–17) μmol/l
Serum alanine aminotransferase	9 (5–15) IU/l
Serum alkaline phosphatase	860 (0–95) IU/l

Figures in parentheses indicate normal ranges.

a) Give two possible causes for the raised alkaline phosphatase level.

b) What investigation would you arrange next?

The sources of a raised alkaline phosphatase level are either liver or bone. The uterus can also make large amounts when it is growing during pregnancy. Always remember to think of these different sources.

CAUSES OF A RAISED ALKALINE PHOSPHATASE

- Biliary obstruction, cholangiocarcinoma, and alcoholic liver disease
- Pregnancy, growing children, Paget's disease
- Temporal arteritis
- Metastatic bone disease, vitamin D deficiency, etc.

Thus, in a young person such as this, a raised alkaline phosphatase may be part of the normal growth spurt associated with puberty. However, in this particular case with the history of weight gain with nausea, the possibility of uterine-derived alkaline phosphatase should be investigated. The membership examiners like a pragmatic approach to the examination and simple answers are often worth the most marks.

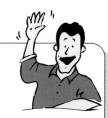

A37
a) Possible causes
Pregnancy or part of normal growth
b) Investigations
Pregnancy test. Abdominal ultrasound.
Ask the patient about the possibility of pregnancy

Q38 A 50-year-old market data manager presents to her casualty with pain in her hips and increasing difficulty standing. She says this has been building up over the last 2 months and that apart from occasional abdominal pain she has noticed nothing else unusual. She has a history of mild hypothyroidism, for which she takes thyroxine. She has no drug allergies although she has recently tried buying different washing powders and soaps as she seems prone to itching. She is a nonsmoker and drinks only socially.

ON EXAMINATION

- Icteric
- Afebrile
- Several bruises over back and upper arms
- Abdominal examination reveals 3 cm hepatomegaly
- Neurological examination reveals 4/5 weakness in the quadriceps muscles

INVESTIGATIONS

- Haemoglobin = 12.4 g/dl
- White cell count = 8.5 x 10⁹/l
- Platelets = 165 x 10⁹/l
- Plasma sodium = 136 mmol/l
- Plasma potassium = 4.5 mmol/l
- Plasma urea = 6.0 mmol/l
- Plasma creatinine = 89 μmol/l
- Plasma calcium = 1.9 mmol/l
- Plasma phosphate = 0.6 mmol/l
- Serum albumin = 38 g/l
- Serum bilirubin = 80 μmol/l
- Serum aspartate aminotransferase = 100 IU/l
- Serum alkaline phosphatase = 850 IU/l
- Prothrombin time = 20 (units)
- APTT = 34 (units)
- Plasma glucose = 5.2 mmol/l

APTT: activated partial thromboplastin time.

a) **What is the underlying diagnosis?**

b) **What one investigation would you do to confirm this?**

c) **What is the cause of her presenting symptoms?**

d) **What management steps would you instigate immediately?**

OK. What are the key abnormal features?

- Obstructive jaundice plus hepatomegaly

- Osteomalacia

- Prolonged prothrombin time

In a middle-aged woman with itching and other evidence of autoimmune disease... you've pretty much got a full house here, short of some weight loss, clubbing, and xanthelasma! If this chick hasn't got primary biliary cirrhosis, then I'm Cleopatra!

A38

a) **Diagnosis**
   Primary biliary cirrhosis

b) **Investigation**
   Antimitochondrial antibodies. Although a liver biopsy is the gold standard test, in this case you would probably lose marks as the patient has a clotting disorder due to malabsorption of vitamin K

c) **Cause of symptoms**
   Osteomalacia due to malabsorption of vitamin D (another fat-soluble vitamin)

d) **Immediate management**
   Calcium and vitamin D supplements
   Correct clotting with intravenous vitamin K

MORE ABOUT PRIMARY BILIARY CIRRHOSIS

Other extra-hepatic features of primary biliary cirrhosis, which may be thrown in to confuse you, are:

- arthralgia
- connective tissue diseases; 75% have Sjögren's syndrome or limited systemic sclerosis
- renal disease: membranous glomerulonephritis or renal tubular acidosis
- cholecystitis: don't forget that people with primary biliary cirrhosis are more prone to pigment gallstones
- dermatitis or neuropathy related to malabsorption of vitamin E

EXTRA BITS: DIFFERENTIAL DIAGNOSIS OF OSTEOMALACIA

EFFECT	CAUSE
Lack of vitamin D	Poor diet Low sun exposure
Vitamin D malabsorption	Postgastrectomy, small bowel surgery, coeliac disease Biliary disease, such as primary biliary cirrhosis (vitamins A, D, E, and K are fat-soluble)
Renal disease	Chronic renal failure Vitamin D-resistant rickets (due to reduced renal tubular phosphate reabsorption) All causes of renal tubular acidosis (proximal and distal)
Miscellaneous	Phenytoin-induced osteomalacia Sclerosing haemangiomas Hypophosphataemic rickets End-organ resistance to 1,25-dihydroxy-vitamin D

Remember:

- Type I hereditary vitamin D-dependent rickets is caused by mutations of the 1α-hydroxylase receptor in the kidneys and responds to physiological quantities of 1,25- dihydroxy-vitamin D
- Type II hereditary vitamin D-dependent rickets is due to mutations in the 1,25-dihydroxy-vitamin D receptor. Some patients may respond to very high doses of 1,25-dihydroxy-vitamin D
- Familial hypophosphataemic (vitamin D-resistant) rickets is an X-linked dominant disorder with low plasma phosphate
- Type I disease has low plasma levels of 1,25-dihydroxy-vitamin D; the other two diseases have high endogenous levels because of end-organ resistance

Q39 A 30-year-old nurse returned to the UK after travelling in the Far East for 8 months. Whilst in Thailand, she received a course of co-trimoxazole for *Shigella* dysentery. Two days after her return flight from Bangkok, she developed abdominal cramping pains with distension and flatulence. She also developed blood-less diarrhoea, which, although initially quite mild, became pale, foul smelling, and difficult to flush away over the course of 2–3 weeks. Her flat-mates took her to casualty, as they were increasingly worried about her poor appetite and the fact that she had lost a considerable amount of weight since her return.

ON EXAMINATION

- Thin, dehydrated and with increased pigmentation on arms and feet
- Weight = 46 kg (previously 51 kg)
- Temperature = 36.6°C
- No clubbing, lymphadenopathy
- Pulse = 110 beats/min regular
- Blood pressure = 95/60 mm Hg
- Cardiovascular examination normal
- Respiratory examination normal
- Abdominal examination: active bowel sounds, nil else

INVESTIGATIONS

- Haemoglobin = 11.5 g/dl
- Plasma sodium = 143 mmol/l
- Plasma potassium = 4.0 mmol/l
- Serum albumin = 28 g/l
- Serum bilirubin = 8 μmol/l
- Plasma urea = 8.2 mmol/l
- White cell count = 6.5 x 10⁹/l
- Platelets = 410 x 10⁹/l
- Rigid sigmoidoscopy = normal
- Faecal fat = 120 mmol/l
- Urinalysis unremarkable

a) Select the three most likely diagnoses:

- tropical sprue
- strongyloidiasis
- gastrointestinal lymphoma
- giardiasis
- adult coeliac disease
- amoebiasis
- persistent shigellosis

b) Select the three appropriate investigations to confirm these:

- barium meal and follow-through
- stool microscopy for ova, cysts, and parasites
- abdominal X-ray
- jejunal biopsy
- duodenal aspirate and biopsy
- abdominal ultrasound
- small bowel enema

We know that the patient has:

- systemic symptoms (weight loss, anorexia, tachycardia)

- textbook malabsorption (steatorrhoea, high faecal fat, blood-less diarrhoea)

The causes of malabsorption have been learned before. Write them down...

Now check them against the picture below:

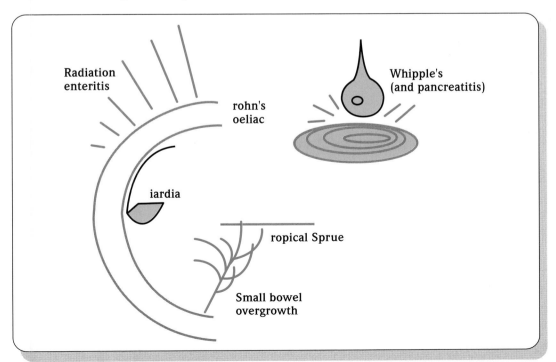

Small bowel lymphoma is also a cause. The tendency is to think of exotic diseases. However, both amoebiasis and shigellosis are associated with bloody diarrhoea, and do not usually cause classic small bowel malabsorption, which is why they do not appear on the list. The same applies to strongyloidiasis, particularly as there is no preceding history of either skin or pulmonary involvement.

From the list, gastrointestinal lymphoma is unlikely without more systemic upset. The same is true for Crohn's disease, particularly as there is an absence of other pointers from the examiner in this direction.

All three remaining diagnoses – giardiasis, tropical sprue, and coeliac disease – have very similar initial presentations but, given the history of recent travel, giardiasis and tropical sprue are the most likely. One would have to exclude these before making a diagnosis of adult coeliac disease.

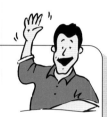

A39

a) Likely diagnoses
Tropical sprue (postinfective tropical malabsorption)
Giardiasis
Adult coeliac disease

b) Investigations
Jejunal biopsy
Stool microscopy for ova, cysts, and parasites
Duodenal aspirate and biopsy

SCHILLING TEST

An alternative strategy that is increasingly being used in the assessment of tropical sprue is to perform a Schilling test, which shows a low vitamin B_{12} uptake in the presence of tropical sprue, then treat with a short course of antibiotics and repeat the Schilling. In tropical sprue, vitamin B_{12} uptake should improve after antibiotic treatment.

Q40

A 30-year-old nurse returned to the UK after travelling in the Far East for 8 months. Whilst in Thailand, she received a course of co-trimoxazole for *Shigella* dysentery. Two days after her return flight from Bangkok, she developed cramping abdominal pains and distension, associated with an itchy rash on her back and feet. She also developed blood-less diarrhoea, which although initially quite mild, became pale, foul smelling, and difficult to flush away over the course of 2–3 weeks. Her flat-mates took her to casualty, as they were increasingly worried about her poor appetite and the fact that she had lost a considerable amount of weight since her return.

ON EXAMINATION

- Thin, dehydrated and with increased pigmentation on arms and feet
- Vesicular rash on back and extensor surfaces
- Angular stomatitis with intra-oral ulceration
- Weight = 46 kg (previously 51 kg)
- Temperature = 36.6°C
- No clubbing, lymphadenopathy
- Pulse = 110 beats/min regular
- Blood pressure = 95/60 mm/Hg
- Cardiovascular examination = normal
- Respiratory examination = normal
- Abdominal examination: active bowel sounds, nil else

INVESTIGATIONS

- Haemoglobin = 9.5 g/dl
- Mean corpuscular volume = 105 fl
- Vitamin B_{12} = 400 pg/ml
- Plasma sodium = 143 mmol/l
- Plasma potassium = 4.0 mmol/l
- Serum albumin = 28 g/l
- Serum bilirubin = 8 μmol/l
- Plasma urea = 8.2 mmol/l
- Plasma creatinine = 115 μmol/l
- White cell count = 6.5 x 10^9/l
- Platelets = 210 x 10^9/l
- Rigid sigmoidoscopy = normal
- Faecal fat = 120 mmol/l
- Urinalysis unremarkable

a) **What is the diagnosis?**

b) **How would you confirm your suspicions?**

c) **What two therapeutic measures would you initiate?**

A very similar question to the previous one! She has:

- systemic features: weight loss, anorexia, tachycardia, mouth ulcers
- malabsorption: steatorrhoea, high faecal fat, macrocytic anaemia – probably due to folate loss
- vesicular, itchy rash on extensor surfaces – dermatitis herpetiformis

In this case, the examiner has given you a strong clue. The presence of dermatitis herpetiformis makes coeliac disease the most likely diagnosis.

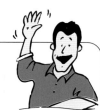

A40

a) **Diagnosis**
   Adult coeliac disease

b) **Investigations**
   Jejunal biopsy to show sub-total villous atrophy
   Antiendomysial IgA antibodies (90% sensitive and specific for coeliac disease)
   Antigliadin antibodies (more sensitive but less specific than antiendomysial)

c) **Therapeutic measures**
   Initiate gluten-free diet
   Give dapsone for the itchy rash of dermatitis herpetiformis. (Note that dapsone causes haemolysis in glucose 6 phosphate dehydrogenase deficiency, methaemoglobinaemia, and peripheral neuropathy)

EXTRA BITS: COELIAC DISEASE

Coeliac disease can crop up in the MRCP examination in a number of disguises.

Cancers

- small/large bowel adenocarcinomas
- small bowel T-cell lymphoma

Diarrhoea/weight loss

- plus mixed blood film: folate and iron-deficiency anaemia
- plus hyposplenic picture: Howell–Jolly bodies, target cells – Pappenheimer bodies, acanthocytes
- plus malabsorption of fat-soluble vitamins:
  - A – visual disturbance
  - D – osteomalacia
  - E – dermatitis, neuropathy
  - K – bleeding, bruising
- plus tetany – a rare complication of coeliac disease
- plus neurological disturbance (long-tract signs and cerebellar ataxia; rare again)
- plus other autoimmune diseases (beware the patient with life-long insulin-dependent diabetes mellitus!)

Q41

A 60-year-old woman presented with sharp epigastric pain that was worse on lying down. This was accompanied by regurgitation of a greenish foul liquid. After 2 weeks of treatment with an H_2 antagonist, her symptoms remained unchanged. Her only other past history was of an underactive thyroid gland for which she took thyroxine 50 μg daily.

ON EXAMINATION

- High body mass index
- Clinical anaemia

INVESTIGATIONS

- Haemoglobin = 9.5 g/dl
- Mean corpuscular volume = 108 fl
- White cell count = 6.5 x 10^9/l
- Platelets = 180 x 10^9/l
- Schilling test without intrinsic factor: urinary radioactive cobalamin excretion = 2%
- Schilling test with intrinsic factor: urinary radioactive cobalamin excretion = 13%

a) **What is the diagnosis?**

b) **What is the cause of her symptoms?**

Again, this is a 'case you should know', rather than a list question. The essence here is that she has:

- vitamin B_{12} deficiency anaemia due to lack of intrinsic factor

- evidence of autoimmune disease (hypothyroidism)

- oesophagitis unresponsive to antacids

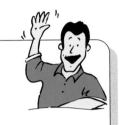

A41 **a) Diagnosis**
Pernicious anaemia

b) Symptom cause
Bile oesophagitis (a feature of pernicious anaemia)

MORE ABOUT PERNICIOUS ANAEMIA

As pernicious anaemia has such an insidious onset, this question comes in a variety of forms:

- the elderly woman with megaloblastic anaemia and peripheral sensory neuropathy

- the patient with autoimmune disease, painful glossitis, and ataxia (due to dorsal column disease)

- the patient with vitiligo, and any of the above factors

QUICK CHECK

Write the lists of causes of:

- bloody diarrhoea

- loss of ankle jerks and upgoing plantars

- eosinophilia

- pyoderma gangrenosum

- cerebrospinal fluid lymphocytosis

And the features of:

- Gilbert's syndrome, Crigler–Najjar syndrome, Dubin–Johnson syndrome

- Friedreich's ataxia

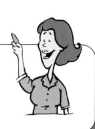

Q42

A 65-year-old woman presents with hip pain and jaundice. She has had intermittent spells of jaundice and abdominal pain for the last 3 years.

INVESTIGATIONS	RESULTS
Haemoglobin	9.8 g/dl
White cell count	3.9 x 10⁹/l
Platelets	179 x 10⁹/l
Serum calcium	1.9 mmol/l
Serum phosphate	0.7 mmol/l
Serum albumin	32 g/l
Serum alanine aminotransferase	7 (5–15) IU/l
Serum alkaline phosphatase	350 (0–95) IU/l
Serum bilirubin	32 (3–17) μmol/l
Clotting INR	1.4
Thrombin time	Normal
Abdominal ultrasound	Normal
Liver biopsy	Liver granulomas with copper deposition

INR: international normalised ratio. Figures in parentheses indicate normal ranges.

a) What is the most likely diagnosis for her jaundice?

b) What test would you do to confirm this diagnosis?

c) What is the cause of her low calcium?

The causes of liver granulomata on biopsy are:

- primary biliary cirrhosis

- classic granulomatous disease: sarcoidosis, TB, Wegener's granulomatosis, *Brucella*, berylliosis

- other autoimmune diseases: IBD., polyarteritis nodosa, giant cell arteritis

- infections? T^2AG along and C^4: tropical (leprosy, schistosomiasis), toxocariasis, ascariasis, giardiasis, *Coxiella*, cytomegalovirus, coccidiodomycosis, clap (syphilis)

- malignancies, drugs, and the chronic granulomatous diseases

The answer ought to scream out at you from this list.

This is a classic membership question that can appear in many formats. Given that the patient has intermittent jaundice with a raised alkaline phosphatase, you should immediately be alerted to this diagnosis. The question has been deliberately made easy by the liver biopsy result. The mention of copper deposition is meant to fool you into diagnosing Wilson's disease (in which granulomata are not seen – see question 23, page 110).

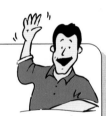

A42 a) **Likely diagnosis**
Primary biliary cirrhosis

b) **Test**
Antimitochondrial antibody/endoscopic retrograde cholangiopancreatography

c) **Low calcium cause**
Osteomalacia (coeliac disease is associated with primary biliary cirrhosis)

QUIZ SPOT!

SIADH CIRCLE

Fill in the letters for four causes of SIADH. If right, the shaded circles will complete a well-known seaside phrase. The solution is on page 252.

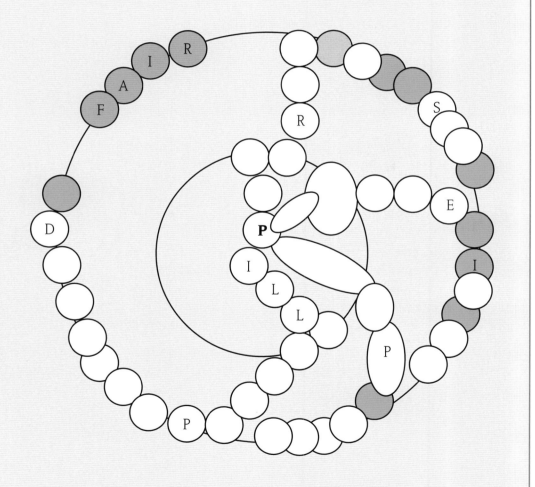

8

A BLOODY HELL

HAEMATOLOGICAL MRCP LISTS

Abnormal haematological results or findings in the reticuloendothelial system are often the key to grey cases and data interpretation questions. If you know nothing else, you must know your haematology lists.

Seen any good films lately?

Top haematology songs

1) You're So Vein (Carly Simon)
2) Lady in Red (Chris de Burr Cell)
3) Whiter Shade of Pale (Procul Harum)

Top haematology films

Any MRCP candidate should know these backwards

1) The Three Colours Trilogy (Red, Blue, and White)
2) Marrowed to the Mob
3) The Cell
4) Spurtigo
5) *Leucoerythroblastosis*
6) *Pancytopenia*
7) *Neutropenia*
8) *Thrombocytopenia*
9) *Polycythaemia*
10) *Eosinophilia*

Reviews of the latter six of the best can be found in this chapter.

Q43

You are asked to see a 6-year-old maladjusted child in a residential home. He presents with a 2-week history of decreasing visual acuity on the right side with the recent onset of blurring of the right eye. Examination reveals the presence of enlarged axillary and cervical lymph nodes. Fundoscopy shows white macular plaques with some retinal detachment.

INVESTIGATIONS	RESULTS
Haemoglobin	11.4 g/dl
White cell count	$6.5 \times 10^9/l$
Eosinophils	20%
Platelets	$156 \times 10^9/l$

a) What is the most likely diagnosis?

b) What three investigations would you do next?

This question is pretty straightforward, using the method we have described. There is only one major list to know, and that is for the causes of eosinophilia. We have done this before (see Pants chapter, page 56): eosinophilia. Try writing down the causes, then check against the list over the page.

CAUSES OF EOS⁴I³N³OP⁶HI⁵LIA

Skin: Rheumatoid arthritis (RA) with cutaneous manifestations

Dermatitis herpetiformis

Scabies

Atopic eczema

Immune: Asthma

Atopy

Any drug reactions

Neoplastic: Hodgkin's lymphomas

Acute lymphoblastic lymphoma

All solid malignancies

Pulmonary: Increases in sputum and peripheral blood eosinophil counts are caused by:

- allergic bronchopulmonary aspergillosis (asthma, cough, sputum plugs, proximal bronchiectasis)
- Löffler's syndrome (cough, fever, yellow sputum, malaise, fluffy X-ray infiltrates)
- tropical eosinophilia (microfilaraemia, ascariasis, ankylostomiasis, toxocariasis, strongyloidiasis)
- drug reactions (co-trimoxazole, busulphan, methotrexate, nitrofurantoin, or anything at all!)
- Churg–Strauss syndrome (small/medium-vessel vasculitis, asthma, eosinophilia)
- adult asthma

Infective: Nematodes – roundworms (e.g. *Toxocara, Ascaris lumbricoides*)

Cestodes – tapeworms (e.g. *Echinococcus*)

Trematodes – flukes

Schistosoma and other parasites

Whipple's disease

You now need to sift through and see which one fits best with the history. With the added recurrent eye problems with retinal detachment and retinal plaques then, against your better judgement, it is time to come up with a weird and wonderful diagnosis. In this case, you can exclude nearly all of them, leaving one major lead contender – and that is *Toxocara* infection.

The additional investigations are difficult. However, in the membership examination, if you suggest an infectious disease as a potential cause of anything then we would recommend going for serology. Given that the patient has **enlarged** lymph nodes then a biopsy is always indicated (a fine needle aspiration is also acceptable).

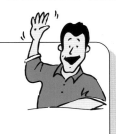

> # A43
> **a) Diagnosis:**
> *Toxocara*
> **b) Investigations:**
> *Toxocara* serology
> *Toxocara* antibodies in the aqueous humour
> Liver, cervical, or axillary node biopsy

T. canis (puppy poo in soil) causes visceral larva migrans, spreading via haematogenous or lymphatic routes to all organs. Systemic inflammation, eosinophilia, itch, breathlessness, and an enlarged liver are all seen, and all the usual features of end-organ inflammation of, for example, brain, lung, and heart. *T. canis* infection is treated with antiparasitic drugs, such as albendazole, usually in combination with anti-inflammatory medications.

LEUCOERYTHROBLASTIC FILM

Immature erythroid and myeloid stem cells appear in the peripheral blood film. This is most commonly due to marrow infiltration causing 'overspill', in which case a high erythrocyte sedimentation rate, normochromic, normocytic anaemia with anisopoikilocytosis, and raised white cell count shift to the left are seen. Alternatively, it may be due to a sudden 'switch on' and outpouring from a marrow 'on the roll'.

M^{5}ARROW INFILTRATIO^{1}NS^3 (OR 'M^{5}O^{1}SS GROWS FAST ON ROLLING BONE')

Causes of leucoerythroblastic film

- Metastases
- Malignancies: myeloma, myeloid leukaemias (chronic myeloid leukaemia and acute myeloid leukaemia)
- Myelofibrosis
- Myeloproliferative (polycythaemia rarely)
- Mycobacteria: tuberculosis (TB)
- Osteopetrosis and Paget's disease
- Sarcoidosis
- Storage: Gaucher's disease – a recessive β-glucocerebrosidase deficiency causing glucocerebroside accumulation, and hence cutaneous pigmentation, hypersplenism, splenomegaly, skeletal deformity. Niemann–Pick disease – autosomal recessive, hepatosplenomegaly, hypersplenism.

Switch on

Massive sepsis, massive haemolysis, or massive haemorrhage leads to pancytopenia.

Causes of pancytopenia

'VD that c²lim⁵bs¹ p¹retty f¹ast'

- **v**iral infections, **d**rug reactions*
- **t**hymic tumours, **h**ypersplenism**, **a**lcohol, **T**B
- **c**arcinoma/**c**hemotherapy, **l**ymphoproliferative disease, **i**rradiation, **m**yelofibrosis, **m**ultiple **m**yeloma, **m**egaloblastic anaemia, **m**yelodysplasia, *Brucella*, **s**ystemic lupus erythematosus (SLE) and **s**ideroblastic anaemia
- **p**aroxysmal nocturnal haemoglobinuria (PNH), **p**arvovirus with sickle cell/haemolytic disease
- **F**anconi's syndrome***, **F**elty's syndrome****

*   Drug reactions can be divided into:

PROPORTIONAL TO DOSE	IDIOSYNCRATIC
Benzene	Sulphonamides/streptomycin
TNT (2,4,6-trinitrotoluene)	Gold/penicillamine/phenoxybenzamine
6-mercaptopurine	Hydralazine
Busulphan	Arsenic
	Acetazolamide
	DDT (dichloro-diphenyl-trichloroethane)

**   See 'Causes of hypersplenism' list, on the next page

***   Fanconi's syndrome: hyperpigmentation, mental retardation, microcephaly, short stature, small thumb/radius/carpus, microsomia, cryptorchidism, hypogonadism

****   Felty's syndrome: splenomegaly, lymphadenopathy, cutaneous pigmentation/ulcers, stomal ulcers in the presence of rheumatoid factor-positive arthritis

CAUSES OF HYPERSPLENISM

6 infections:
- TB
- *Brucella*
- syphilis
- malaria
- subacute bacterial endocarditis (SBE)
- kala azar

6 haematological:
- lymphoma
- chronic lymphocytic leukaemia (CLL)
- chronic myelocytic leukaemia (CML)
- myelofibrosis
- thalassaemia/haemoglobinopathies
- haemolysis

5 autoimmune:
- RA
- Still's disease
- Felty's syndrome
- SLE
- pernicious anaemia

4 other:
- congestion
- sarcoidosis
- amyloidosis
- idiopathic

3 blanks

2 metabolic:
- Gaucher's disease
- Niemann–Pick disease

ANSWERS TO CRITERIA CONNECTIONS (see page 16): You need two major criteria, or one major and at least two minor, to make the diagnosis. Missing are: past rheumatic fever (minor), and arthralgia (minor, if polyarthropathy absent).

Causes of neutropenia

That may seem a lot to learn, but you can use this list as the basis for another list. You might have thought that PIES[2] could cause bovine spongiform encephalitis (BSE). But who would have thought that they were the cause of *neutropenia*?

Pancytopenia: all causes in the list above

Infection: typhoid, typhus, TB, any type of viral infection, *Brucella*, kala azar, malaria

Endocrine: hypopituitarism, and both hypothyroidism and hyperthyroidism

SLE

Specific drugs: alcohol and alcoholic cirrhosis, thiouracil

Causes of thrombocytopenia

The causes are really pretty straightforward:

* the causes of neutropenia
* consumption in clots (disseminated intravascular coagulation), by the spleen (hypersplenism including Felty's syndrome), and by autoimmune mechanisms (idiopathic thrombocytopenic purpura)
* dilution (massive transfusion)
* marrow invasion or toxic suppression

Causes of polycythaemia

We're bored now. Make up your own way of remembering the causes. Here they are:

Relative: dehydration

                         Gaisböck's syndrome (stress)

Primary: polycythaemia rubra vera (splenomegaly, raised platelets)

Secondary: hypoxia, chronic obstructive pulmonary disease, altitude, abnormal haemoglobin, sleep apnoea

Excess erythropoietin: cerebellar haemangioma

                         hepatoma

                         phaeochromocytoma

                         hypernephroma

                         polycystic/transplant kidneys

                         uterine leiomyomata/fibromata

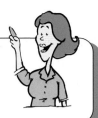

Q44

What do target cells, Howell–Jolly bodies, siderocytes, microspherocytes, and a high platelet and neutrophil count signify?

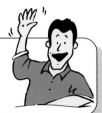

A44

Hyposplenism. Learn these features – it a common finding in the MRCP examination and can crop up in a number of different guises.

FASCINATING FACT

Auer rods are seen in acute promyelocytic leukaemia (PML) as rod-shaped inclusions in white blood cells. Not many people wanted to know that.

SIZE AND SHAPE DO MATTER

Sorry. But they do. Of course they do, and nowhere more so than in the haematology question. You can get clues to the diagnosis of short and grey cases by looking for abnormal features of the red blood cells.

Macrocytosis

Macrocytosis is a common finding that usually represents the release into the circulation of immature (and therefore large) red blood cell precursors. Most candidates can think of very few causes – namely liver disease and vitamin B_{12} deficiency. Pause here, and write yourself a list of 15 other causes. When you have finally had enough, learn the list below:

L^3EG CR^{3}A^{3}M^{4}P^{2}S^1 = 17

- liver disease, leukoerythroblastosis, lead poisoning
- cytotoxic chemotherapy
- reticulocytosis, renal failure, respiratory failure
- alcohol ingestion, aplastic anaemia, azathioprine treatment
- megaloblastic anaemia (vitamin B_{12}/folate deficiency), myeloma, myxoedema, malaria
- pregnancy, pellagra
- sideroblastic anaemia

Spherocytosis

Spherocytes have a round, uniform shape, just as their name suggests. As usual, this finding can be hereditary or acquired. As a rule of thumb, *structural defects* are usually *dominant*, and *metabolic* defects are usually *recessive*. Thus, hereditary spherocytosis (a structural defect caused by *defects* in membrane stabilising proteins) is transmitted as an autosomal dominant condition and is not associated with haemolysis. However, just like injured cattle, injured red blood cells are rounded up. Thus, any red blood cell injury can cause haemolysis, and all causes of haemolysis can produce spherocytes.

Target cells

Take the stuffing out of a cushion and sit on it and it will look like a target. Similarly, any very thin red blood cell will look like a target. How do you knock the stuffing out of a red blood cell? Quite simply by mucking up its haemoglobin. The causes are, therefore, sickle cell disease, sickle/haemoglobin C, haemoglobin C disease, haemoglobin C/thalassaemia, thalassaemia (major and minor), and iron deficiency. Simple isn't it? Oh, by the way, post-splenectomy patients may also have target cells.

Howell–Jolly bodies

These are tiny granules of damaged DNA in red blood cells. Normally the spleen would filter out these cells. Thus, you see them when the spleen isn't there (i.e. in *any cause of hyposplenism*, including post-splenectomy and sickle cell disease), or when the spleen is overwhelmed with damaged cells, such as in haemolysis, toxic anaemias, and the lymphoid leukaemias.

Siderocytes

These contain granules of nonhaemoglobin iron (Pappenheimer bodies), which stain blue at the edge of the cell with Wright stain. Think metals (haemochromatosis, lead poisoning), prematurity, pernicious anaemia, thalassaemia, myelodysplasia/proliferation, and haemolysis. It may also be caused by RA and some drugs (e.g. chloramphenicol). The most common cause, however, is alcoholism.

We can't think of an easy way to remember this list. Feel free to try!

MAHA

MAHA, or microangiopathic haemolytic anaemia to its friends, can be recognised by the presence of fragmented red blood cells and burr cells. The causes are:

- growths: cancers, foetuses (eclampsia, abruption, intrauterine death, amniotic fluid embolus)
- damage to small vessels (malignant hypertension, vasculitides, burns, sepsis, and disseminated intravascular coagulation [DIC])
- renal-failure association:
  thrombotic thrombocytopenic purpura (TTP)
  haemolytic uraemic syndrome (HUS)
  acute glomerulonephritis
- drugs: such as cytotoxics, cyclosporin.

Note that TTP is another name for Moschcowitz disease. This is the same as HUS, but with added fever, neurological impairment, and mild abnormalities of clotting with haemolysis and renal impairment. It is associated with infection (especially verotoxin-producing *Escherichia coli*), SLE, and cancers. Remember that the causes of MAHA overlap with those of standard haemolytic anaemia.

Causes of haemolytic anaemia

We couldn't think of a funny mnemonic for these, but the causes are relatively well known so we will just list them. If you can come up with something that is amusing then we would be pleased to hear from you.

Congenital

- Membrane defects: hereditary spherocytosis/elliptocytosis
- Haemoglobinopathies: sickle cell anaemia, thalassaemia
- Enzyme problems: glucose-6-phosphate dehydrogenase deficiency, pyruvate kinase deficiency

Acquired

- Immune: autoimmune, lymphoma, RA, drug induced (e.g. methyldopa, penicillin), post-transfusion, PNH
- MAHA: mechanical injury, malaria, prosthetic valves, burns, clostridial sepsis *(Clostridium perfringens)*, snake bites, march haemoglobinuria
- DIC
- Hypersplenism

Remember that hyposplenic patients, particularly children, are susceptible to infections with *Klebsiella, E. coli, Streptococcus pneumoniae, Haemophilus influenzae* type B (HIB), and *Neisseria meningitidis*. These patients should be given prophylactic penicillin (erythromycin for allergic patients).

HEPATOMEGALY

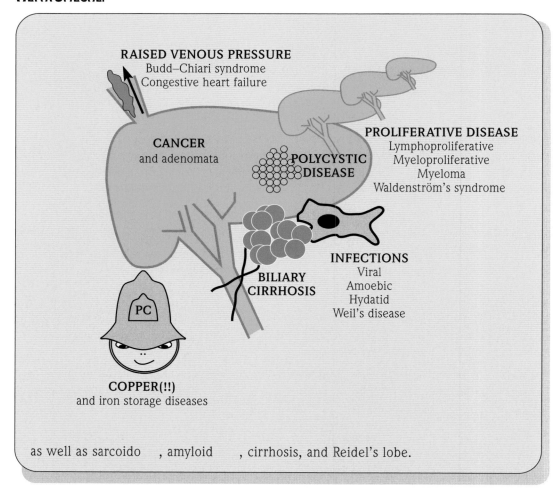

as well as sarcoido , amyloid , cirrhosis, and Reidel's lobe.

Learn to draw the picture above, or invent your own.

Remember that:

- the top three common causes are cirrhosis, congestive heart failure, and malignancy
- hard and knobbly suggests malignancy, cirrhosis (particularly after hepatitis B infection), polycystic disease, hydatid cyst, or syphilis.

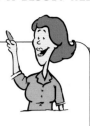

Q45

A 23-year-old man is admitted for the investigation of anaemia. It is noted that he has a palpable spleen. There is no hepatomegaly or lymphadenopathy, and the patient is otherwise well, except that he has recently suffered a mild upper airway infection.

INVESTIGATIONS	RESULTS
Haemoglobin	8.9 g/dl
White cell count	6.5 x 10⁹/l
Platelets	234 x 10⁹/l
Reticulocytes	9%
Spherocytes	Present

a) What three tests would you do to investigate this patient further?

This sort of question is always a good one, and an example of why the MRCP examination is in love with haematology. It's just so easy to mix up a few good clinical signs with a few odd blood tests.

Here we could go for several lists, but the obvious one is for the causes of splenomegaly. Again, try to jot down as complete a list as you can before looking at the summary overleaf.

CAUSES OF SPENOMEGALY

MASSIVE	MODERATE	MILD
• Chronic myeloid leukaemia • Myelofibrosis • Malaria • Kala azar • Gaucher's disease	• All causes of massive splenomegaly • Myeloproliferation • Cirrhosis and portal hypertension • Leukaemia • Haemolysis	• All causes of massive/moderate splenomegaly • Infection • Lymphoproliferative disorders • Immunoproliferative disorders

Other causes

• *Brucella*, typhoid, TB, trypanosomiasis, SBE, viral infections (infectious mononucleosis [IMN], hepatitis B)

• Sarcoidosis, amyloidosis

• SLE, Felty's syndrome

• ITP, haemolysis, iron deficiency, pernicious anaemia

We know that the patient is anaemic with a high reticulocyte count, and must therefore be bleeding or haemolysing. The chances of a young man bleeding *and* having a big spleen are small, unless you want to invoke DIC with a lymphoma, or liver disease with an impalpable liver, no other signs, and portal hypertension. The likelihood is that he is haemolysing – a conclusion you should have reached even without the presence of spherocytes on the film. Now combine the splenomegaly list with the haemolytic anaemia list and... hey presto!

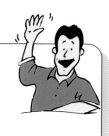

A45 a) **Tests**
Coomb's test
Glucose-6-phosphate dehydrogenase level
Red cell pyruvate kinase level
Blood film for spherocytes/elliptocytes
Take a family history

HEPATOSPLENOMEGALY

Well, at last it gets easier. The causes are simply all those of splenomegaly, plus thalassaemia and all the causes of hepatomegaly, with the exception of biliary cirrhosis and proliferative disease.

HEPATOSPLENOMEGALY

Here we hit the **Wall**:

- **W**aldenström's syndrome

- **a**cute lymphoblastic leukaemia

- **l**ymphoma

- (and think of the other **l**ymphoproliferative disorders)

Common tests

ESR THROUGH THE ROOF

Think of:

- first line – temporal arteritis, polymyalgia rheumatica, SLE, multiple myeloma

- second line – carcinoma and chronic infection.

LAP DANCING

What the hell is LAP? OK, so it stands for leucocyte alkaline phosphatase. But a score? I ask you! OK, if you *really* want to know… it's found in neutrophils. The earlier the neutrophil precursor or the younger the cell, the higher the LAP score. So anything that causes you to increase the production of young or immature neutrophils will cause a rise in LAP score. Make a list of these causes below, and then check it out against ours.

Causes of high LAP scores
- myeloproliferative disorders: polycythaemia rubra vera, myelofibrosis, Hodgkin's disease
- steroids: Cushing's syndrome, treatment with steroids, the oral contraceptive pill, pregnancy

It is also:
- *up* in *Down's* syndrome
- *up* when protein levels are *down* (e.g. in kwashiorkor when serum levels are low!)

Causes of low LAP scores
LAP score is low in things with letters in:
- chronic myelocytic leukaemia (CML)
- pernicious anaemia (PA)
- IMN or Epstein–Barr virus (EBV)
- paroxysmal nocturnal haemoglobinuria (PNH)

as well as in:
- rickets
- hypophosphataemia

Osmotic fragility

In the presence of an osmotic challenge, some cells are resistant to bursting, and are said to show decreased osmotic fragility. These are best remembered as being the cells with abnormal haemoglobin: haemoglobin C, sickle cells, thalassaemia, iron and vitamin B_{12} deficiency. Increased fragility is seen in all haemolytic states: it is the classic test for spherocytosis.

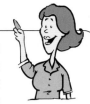

Q46

An 8-year-old girl of Nigerian origin, recently arrived in the UK, presents to her local Accident and Emergency Department with a 10-day history of fever and malaise. She lives with her parents and she has a 5-year-old brother who has been in complete remission from acute lymphoblastic leukaemia (ALL) for 1 year. Her mother is a primary school teacher and her father is in the diplomatic service, necessitating the family to move to different countries twice a year. Ten days before the onset of her symptoms, she had a 1-week course of antibiotics from her GP for a throat infection. In addition to her fever, she complains of several days' pain and swelling in both hands. She has had no gastrointestinal disturbance or overt signs of blood loss. She has had similar attacks before.

ON EXAMINATION

- Temperature = 37.5°C
- Pulse = 98 beats/min regular
- Blood pressure = 105/70 mmHg
- No rashes or lymphadenopathy
- Mild icterus
- Mouth clear
- Jugular venous pressure not elevated
- Heart sounds 1+2+soft ejection systolic murmur left sternal edge
- Chest clear
- Abdomen soft, no hepatosplenomegaly
- Painful dactylitis of the right index and ring fingers, and the left middle and ring fingers

INVESTIGATIONS

- Haemoglobin = 9.0 g/l
- Reticulocytes = 8%
- White cell count = 13 x 10⁹/l
- Neutrophils = 85%
- Platelets = 450 x 10⁹/l
- Urinalysis and electrolytes = normal
- Bilirubin = 40 μmol/l
- Aspartate aminotransferase = 45 IU/l
- ESR = 130 mm in the first hour
- CRP = 76 mg/l
- Urinalysis: normal dipstick, no casts/cells, negative cultures
- ECG: sinus rhythm, PR interval 0.18 s, QRS 0.12 s, QT 0.4 s, normal axis

CRP: C-reactive protein; ECG: electrocardiogram; ESR: erythrocyte sedimentation rate.

a) **The most likely diagnosis is:**
- polyarticular Still's disease
- acute rheumatic fever
- hand-and-foot syndrome of sickle cell disease
- Lyme disease

b) **Which one investigation will confirm your diagnosis?**
- antinuclear antibody and autoantibody screen
- haemoglobin electrophoresis
- rheumatoid factor
- blood cultures
- acute and convalescent serum antistreptolysin O titres
- left knee aspiration, microscopy, and culture
- anti-*Borrelia burgdorferi* IgM antibody

c) **What is the appropriate management? (select three)**
- corticosteroid therapy
- nonsteroidal anti-inflammatory drugs
- bed rest
- blood transfusion
- penicillamine
- physiotherapy
- family screening and counselling
- opiate analgesia

You have seen a similar question before (at least we hope that you can recognise it!) – in the Strategy chapter. The history here, however, is slightly different: in this case there is a preceding infection followed by a painful dactylitis of the hands and haemolytic anaemia in a younger child of African origin. This alone must make sickle cell disease scream out to be diagnosed. But let us suppose that you were blinded by fear in the examination. The key features with a limited list of causes are:

- polyarthralgia in the hands: remind yourself of the causes (AGAIN!) below
- haemolysis or blood loss: again, check that you know these by writing them down.

Causes of polyarthralgia

Causes of haemolysis

The absence of abdominal or bowel symptoms excludes (for the examination) the whole of the last verse of the polyarthralgia poem. None of the first or second verses are associated with anaemia and a *high reticulocyte count* (suggesting haemolysis or blood loss). The last verse is also out. But remember, we had two causes at the bottom that were not part of the verse. We said, 'remember the haematological causes: sickle cell disease, which can give rise to hand-and-foot syndrome'. In addition, 'remember that septic polyarthritis can occur when joints are seeded with organisms such as *Neisseria gonorrhoeae* or *Staphylococcus*'.

This leaves septic polyarthritis (excluded on the same grounds), or sickle cell disease.

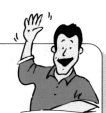

A46

a) **Diagnosis**
Sickle cell disease with hand-and-foot syndrome

b) **Investigation**
Haemoglobin electrophoresis

c) **Management**
Opiate analgesia
Blood transfusion
Family screening and counselling

QUIZ SPOT!

Q: What are the six pulmonary causes of peripheral (circulating) eosinophilia?

A: See page 56 for the list of causes.

Q47 A 30-year-old Caucasian man presents to casualty with a 10-day history of wrist-drop. He did some heavy lifting recently while helping a friend to move house and wonders whether this could have contributed. He suffers from asthma and chronic rhinitis, which are currently well controlled on regular inhaled steroids. On direct questioning he recalls having had foot-drop some years ago, but this was somewhat overshadowed by an acute exacerbation of asthma at the same time, for which he required hospital admission. On his discharge from hospital the foot-drop had resolved and he thought nothing more about it.

ON EXAMINATION

- Looks well apart from obvious left radial nerve palsy, and some adductor weakness of the right thumb. He cannot stand on the tips of his toes
- 3–4 tender subcutaneous nodules on dorsum of arm
- Remainder of examination, including full neurological examination = normal

INVESTIGATIONS

- Skin nodule biopsy shows noncaseating granuloma
- Haemoglobin = 14 g/dl
- White cell count = 12 x 10⁹/l
- Eosinophils = 2.0 x 10⁹/l
- Platelets = 281 x 10⁹/l
- Plasma sodium = 135 mmol/l
- Plasma potassium = 4.9 mmol/l
- Plasma urea = 8.1 mmol/l
- Plasma creatinine = 160 μmol/l

a) **What is the underlying diagnosis?**

b) **What is the mechanism of this patient's wrist-drop?**

c) **What treatment would you start?**

The key features here are:

- eosinophilia
- noncaseating granuloma
- atopic background

You already know the list of causes of eosinophilia (see Pants chapter, page 56).

Causes of eos⁴i³n³op⁶hi⁵lia

Skin: RA with cutaneous manifestations

            Dermatitis herpetiformis

            Scabies

            Atopic eczema

Immune: Asthma

            Atopy

            Any drug reactions

Neoplastic: Hodgkin's lymphomas

            Acute lymphoblastic lymphoma

            All solid malignancies

Pulmonary: Increases in sputum and peripheral blood eosinophil counts are caused by:

- allergic bronchopulmonary aspergillosis (asthma, cough, sputum plugs, proximal bronchiectasis)
- Löffler's syndrome (cough, fever, yellow sputum, malaise, fluffy X-ray infiltrates)
- tropical eosinophilia (microfilaraemia, ascariasis, ankylostomiasis, toxocariasis, strongyloidiasis)
- drug reactions (co-trimoxazole, busulphan, methotrexate, nitrofurantoin, or anything at all!)
- Churg–Strauss syndrome (small/medium-vessel vasculitis, asthma, eosinophilia)
- adult asthma

Infective: Nematodes – roundworms (e.g. *Toxocara, Ascaris lumbricoides*)

            Cestodes – tapeworms (e.g. *Echinococcus*)

            Trematodes – flukes

            Schistosoma and other parasites

            Whipple's disease

CAUSES OF POLYNEUROPATHY

You might want to add in a list of causes of acquired polyneuropathy, which you learned earlier (see page 42).

Born unlucky:	Friedreich's ataxia, Refsum's disease, Charcot–Marie–Tooth disease
Three dejected:	alcoholics due to the effects of alcohol: vitamin B_1, B_6, and B_{12} deficiencies: isoniazid used to treat TB – which is why people receiving TB treatment must receive pyridoxine supplements
Two infected:	leprosy, Guillain–Barré syndrome
Two injected:	paraneoplasia in cancer patients, or the effects of its treatments, such as vincristine and isoniazid; diabetes mellitus
One connected:	connective tissue disease, such as RA/SLE/polyarteritis nodosa
Granuloma suspected:	sarcoidosis, Churg–Strauss syndrome, and hypothyroid

This should leave you with two likely answers; lymphoma or Churg–Strauss syndrome. Only one gives rise to granulomata...

A47

a) **Diagnosis**
Churg–Strauss syndrome

b) **Cause of wrist-drop**
Mononeuritis multiplex

c) **Treatment**
Corticosteroids, reducing the dose over the course of 2 weeks according to symptoms

CHURG–STRAUSS SYNDROME

This is characterised by:

- asthma (typically males in their thirties)
- *medium* vessel vasculitis
- extravascular granulomas
- history of atopy/asthma/rhinitis that usually preceded granuloma

- peripheral blood eosinophilia
- mild renal impairment
- mononeuritis multiplex
- perinuclear antineutrophil cytoplasm antibody (P-ANCA) positive in 50% (as opposed to Wegener's granulomatosis, see below).

WEGENER'S GRANULOMATOSIS

This is characterised by:

- *small* vessel vasculitis
- extravascular granulomas
- any two of upper respiratory, lower respiratory, or renal involvement
- upper respiratory tract: stuffiness, sinusitis, nasal bridge collapse, nasal mucosa granuloma, conductive deafness
- lower respiratory tract: haemoptysis, pulmonary cavitating lesions, pleuritic pain
- renal: acute renal failure, rapidly progressive glomerulonephritis
- occasional but rare involvement of skin and nervous system
- cytoplasmic antineutrophil cytoplasm antibody (C-ANCA) positive

EXTRA BITS: VARIATIONS TO QUESTION

This question may appear in a similar format but with a few changes.

- Young man + wheeze/asthma + eosinophilia + history of ulcerative colitis = eosinophilic alveolitis secondary to sulphasalazine
- Young female + wheeze + eosinophilia + recurrent urinary tract infections = eosinophilic alveolitis secondary to nitrofurantoin

CAUSES OF GRANULOMATA

- Sarcoidosis
- TB (caseating)
- Langerhans cell histiocytosis
- Wegener's granulomatosis
- Churg–Strauss syndrome
- Fungal and helminthic infections
- Hypersensitivity reactions (e.g. dust)
- Malignancy (primary or secondary to colon, kidney, germ-cell, bone, prostate, melanoma)

Q48

A 35-year-old woman is referred to her local gastroenterologist for investigation of recurrent abdominal pain. She denies any diarrhoea, mucus or slime in the stool. (By the way, who would want to be a gastroenterologist?) She is otherwise fit and well apart from having had a left tibial vein thrombosis 3 years ago and a right deep vein thrombosis 8 months ago. On direct questioning she complains of intermittent pain and swelling of her fingers, but this has not been severe enough for her to be worried. On examination she is clinically anaemic, but findings are otherwise unremarkable.

INVESTIGATIONS	RESULTS
Haemoglobin	8.5 g/dl
White cell count	2.1 x 10⁹/l
Platelets	85 x 10⁹/l
Reticulocytes	10%
Serum bilirubin	21 μmol/l
Serum aspartate aminotransferase	16 IU/l
Serum alkaline phosphatase	75 IU/l
Prothrombin time	14 s
Activated partial thromboplastin time	38 s

a) What is the diagnosis?

b) How would you confirm this with only two tests?

This is a 'just know it' question. The key features are:

- recurrent venous thromboses
- pancytopenia (with haemolytic anaemia)
- small joint arthropathy.

You might consult your list of causes of polyarthropathy – it must be on there. Run through the poem and add-ons (see page 5) and the causes are:

- RA, Still's disease, osteoarthritis, seronegative arthritides, pyrophosphate arthropathy, and SLE (Henoch–Schönlein purpura, sarcoidosis, and serum sickness are also included in the poem)
- infections: Parvovirus, *Neisseria gonorrhoeae*, *Streptococcus*, TB, German measles, hepatitis, Lyme disease, chickenpox, HIV, and subacute bacterial endocarditis are also included in the poem
- bowel-associated: familial Mediterranean fever, inflammatory bowel disease, Whipple's disease
- sickle cell anaemia
- Behçets syndrome

Which of these can cause thrombotic tendency? Well, Crohn's disease and ulcerative colitis can. So, too, can SLE (lupus anticoagulant). The absence of altered bowel habit is meant to point you towards SLE.

A48
a) **Diagnosis**
Systemic lupus erythematosus
b) **Tests**
Antinuclear antibodies (very sensitive – 90% positive)
Antibodies to double-stranded DNA (very specific, but only present in 50% of cases)

The abdominal pain is believed to be due to small portal vein occlusions by thromboses.

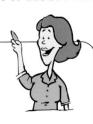

Q49

A 30-year-old man is investigated for recurrent venous thrombosis. Apart from the intermittent passage of dark urine, he is a fit person and regularly plays five-aside football on Saturday mornings.

INVESTIGATIONS	RESULTS
Haemoglobin	9.5 g/dl
White cell count	2.5 x 10^9/l (normal differential)
Reticulocytes	12%
Platelets	90 x 10^9/l

a) What is the diagnosis, and what tests would you perform?

A49 a) **Diagnosis**
This is a classic case. No lists here, then! You just have to know that this is paroxysmal nocturnal haemoglobinuria (PNH). Diagnosis is with Ham's acid lysis/acidified serum test; cells from patients with PNH readily lyse in acidified serum.

Red cells are especially sensitive to complement lysis as pH lowers. Thus, anything that makes the blood more acid (including intense exercise, operative stress, and hypoventilation during sleep) can cause continued intravascular haemolysis. It may be associated with abdominal pain, pancytopenia, all the features of haemolysis (including reticulocytosis and slight jaundice), dark urine (from haemoglobin, often in the morning), and tendency to thrombosis (arterial or venous); hence, sudden ascites and abdominal pain in such a case of PNH with portal vein thrombosis.

Quick refresher

List the causes of:

- cerebellar syndromes
- splenomegaly
- pulmonary eosinophilia

And the causes of:
- spherocytosis
- erythema multiforme
- pancytopenia
- hepatomegaly

ALL IN ONE: EVERYTHING YOU WANTED TO KNOW ABOUT HAEMATOLOGY...

YOU MAY WANT TO CUT THIS OUT AND PUT IT ON YOUR WALL, OR CARRY IT AROUND WITH YOU.

Group	Diagnosis	Liver	Spleen	Nodes	Haematological comments	Other comments to note
Chronic Myeloproliferative disorders	Essential thrombocythaemia	+	+ (leading to atrophy)			LAP high ; Philadelphia chromosome negative; may have high B_{12} and urate
	PVR	+	+		NN anaemia if phlebotomy is prescribed; WCC high in 60%; platelet count high in 50%	LAP high; low iron; high total iron binding capacity; may have high B_{12} and urate
	Myelofibrosis	+	++		May have features of hypersplenism or pancytopenia; WCC high or low; platelet count high or low	LAP high; high SBR concentration and LDH; low folate; may have high B_{12} and urate
	CML	+	++		+/- NN anaemia; WCC high+++; platelet count high or low; neutro++, myelocytes++, blasts++	LAP low; may have high B_{12} and urate
Lymphoproliferative disorders	Prolymphocytic leukaemia		+	(+/-)	Prolymphocytes >100; variant of CLL, but no nodes and a big early spleen	Systemic symptoms +++
	CLL	+	(+/-)	+	Lymphocytosis 100–500; NN anaemia; platelet count low; smear cells with or without haemolysis	Reduced immunoglobulins +/- IgM or light chain band
	Hairy-cell leukaemia	+	+	(+/-)	BM involvement or hypersplenism lead to pancytopenia	
	HMR	+	+		Pancytopenia	
	Infectious mononucleosis	+ (20%)	+ (50%)	+	Lymphocytes <30; platelet count may be low; haemolysis possible	IgM high; cold agglutinin; heterophil antibodies react with beef but not guinea pig; LFT abnormal
	Non-Hodgkin's lymphoma	+	+	+	NN anaemia in 15%–30%; BM involvement; ESR very high; leucoerythroblastic film; lymphocytes+++ (unlike Hodgkin's)	$CaPO_4$ high; urate high; LFT abnormal; acute phase reactants (incl caeruloplasmin) raised
	Hodgkin's lymphoma	+	+	++	Often normal or NN anaemia, lymphopenia: high platelets, ESR, eosinophils, and neutrophils; leucoerythroblastic; less BM involved	$CaPO_4$ high; urate high; LFT abnormal; acute phase reactants (including caeruloplasmin) raised
Acute Leukaemias	Myelodysplastic		+/-	+/-	Pancytopenia with NN anaemia or high MCV; hypergranular cells	
	AML	+/-	+	+/-	WCC <4 in 50%, normal in 20%, high in 30%; NN anaemia; platelets low; Sudan black positive; neutrophil Auer rod positive	Urate high; myelocyte lysozyme raised
	ALL	+	+	++	WCC high (often <10 in children); blasts++; NN anaemia; platelets low	Urate high; sodium may be low; potassium may be low
And not forgetting...	PNH	+/-	+		Pancytopenia with reticulocytosis	Occasional jaundice with haemosiderinuria
	Myeloma	+ (40%)	+ (10%)		NN anaemia leading to pancytopenia; high ESR; rouleaux (except pure light chain); leucoerythroblastic	
	Waldenstrom's	+	+	+		

ALL: acute lymphoblastic leukaemia; AML: acute myeloblastic leukaemia; BM: bone marrow; CLL: chronic lymphocytic leukaemia; CML: chronic myeloid leukaemia; ESR: erythrocyte sedimentation rate; HMR: histiocytic medullary reticulosis; LAP: leucocyte alkaline phosphatase; LDH: lactate dehydrogenase; LFT: liver function tests; MCV: mean corpuscular volume; NN anaemia: normocytic normochromic anaemia; PNH: paroxysmal nocturnal haemoglobinuria; PVR: polycythaemia rubra vera; SBR: serum bilirubin; WCC: white cell count.

9

TAKING THE P**S

RENAL MRCP LISTS

Renal questions are interesting. They usually refer to oliguria or anuria, yet engender almost exactly the opposite sign (immediate loss of sphincter control with subsequent flooding) in most candidates. Renal medicine is actually, however, quite fun in the membership examination, even if not in real life.

Actually scratch all the above – it isn't fun. This is a total lie. It's a pain. Clinical renal medicine involves obtaining urea and creatinine measurements every 2 hours, and nodding in a sage and mature fashion, as if you are really interested in active sediment. The MRCP examination medicine is just as smart-arsed.

However, there are one or two recurrent themes, which tend to revolve around the presence of nephrotic syndrome or glomerulonephritis. Occasional 'casts' are thrown in, but these are usually to confuse.

Nephrotic syndrome appears in a number of guises. The questions revolve around one of three things:

- making the diagnosis of nephrotic syndrome
- identifying the likely cause
- recognising that the findings in grey cases are complications of nephrotic syndrome

In terms of making the diagnosis, provided you are alert to the classical triad of oedema, hypoalbuminaemia, and proteinuria (defined by a urinary protein level $>3.5 \text{ g}/1.73 \text{ m}^2$ of body surface area per day) you shouldn't get caught out. Causes are best remembered by the following verse.

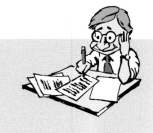

NEPHROTIC SYNDROME

SBE and SLE
RA treatment[†] – cloudy pee
Murky water in the area?
Think, as ever, of malaria.

Amyloid and sickle too
Piss neat protein down the loo.
Remember, too, that cancer* can
Give frothy urine in the PAN.

Nephrotic diabetic piss
Isn't something one should miss
With water, sugar, protein – think
It makes a fortifying drink!

[†] gold, penicillamine, nonsteroidal anti-inflammatory drugs (NSAIDs), captopril, interferon-α, and heroin
*especially lymphoma
Amyloid: amyloidosis; PAN: polyarteritis nodosa; RA: rheumatoid arthritis; SBE: subacute bacterial endocarditis; sickle: sickle cell disease; SLE: systemic lupus erythematosus

Other rare causes include bee stings. Renal vein thrombosis is also a cause, as is pre-eclampsia. Infectious causes include HIV, hepatitis B/C, syphilis, and parasites, such as schistosomiasis. Despite the verse above, glomerulonephritis is the underlying cause of nephrotic syndrome in 80% of cases.

Finally, cases are sometimes dressed up by presentation with one of the complications of nephrotic syndrome, which are th^{2}romb^{2}oti^{3}c:

- thrombosis
- hyperlipidaemia, hyponatraemia
- renal vein thrombosis
- osteomalacia
- malnutrition
- B$_{12}$ deficiency, Budd–Chiari syndrome
- iron deficiency, infection, immunodeficiency.

As we have said, the commonest cause of nephrotic syndrome is actually glomerulonephritis, and this diagnosis itself has many potential causes; glomerulonephritis is always a tricky issue. Here, therefore, is a quick summary.

IgA GLOMERULONEPHRITIS/BERGER'S DISEASE

- Histology: mesangial expansion/hypercellularity (hyperplasia)
- Aetiology: unknown – possible IgA dysregulation and abnormal sialidation (glycosylation)
- Associations: cirrhosis; dermatitis herpetiformis; gluten-enteropathy; mycosis fungoides (T-cell lymphoma); other malignancies; ankylosing spondylitis; Wiskott–Aldrich syndrome; chronic liver/lung disease; human leucocyte antigen (HLA) DQW7/B35
- Epidemiology: the commonest primary glomerulonephritis. Increased incidence in the Far East and in men
- Presentation: varied: microscopic or macroscopic haematuria triggered by prodromal infection (upper respiratory tract infection [URTI]); proteinuria or overt nephrotic syndrome; rapidly progressive glomerulonephritis with crescents; hypertension; chronic renal failure
- Prognosis: 20% develop end-stage renal failure after 20 years. Prognosis is better in those who initially present with episodic macroscopic haematuria, well-controlled blood pressure and little proteinuria
- Treatment:
  - asymptomatic – leave alone
  - mild disease – fish oils
  - acute nephritis (rapidly progressing glomerulonephritis [RPGN]) – possibly immunosuppression with cyclophosphamide, corticosteroids and plasma exchange

Minimal change glomerulonephritis

- Histology: normal under light microscopy ('minimal change'!), but epithelial foot process effacement under electron microscopy; selective proteinuria
- Aetiology: unknown, possibly immune
- Associations: HLA B12; URTIs; vaccinations; Hodgkin's disease; rifampicin; NSAIDs; gold; Epstein–Barr virus/HIV; atopy; obesity; heroin; Fabry's disease; sialidosis
- Epidemiology: the commonest primary cause of nephrotic syndrome in children (90%) and causes 20%–30% of nephrotic syndrome cases in adults
- Presentation: nephrotic syndrome; hyperlipidaemia; acute renal failure, especially if volume-depleted
- Prognosis: very good in children; most are steroid-responsive; thus, biopsy is only indicated when disease is unresponsive to steroids, when cyclosporin can be used. In adults, about 40% of cases are steroid-responsive and, as there is a spectrum of other diseases causing nephrotic syndrome, they should all be biopsied.

Focal segmental glomerulosclerosis

This is characterised by accumulation of hyaline/proteinaceous material in parts (segments) of glomeruli, affecting less than 50% of glomeruli in any given biopsy. Many nephrologists feel that this is an advanced form of minimal change disease that has progressed to protein deposition and glomerular distortion. Aetiologically, it arises from a similar range of factors as minimal change disease and other sustained protein deposition in the kidneys. It is as if the kidneys have been chronically exposed to a clogging influence and the filter is dirty. Again, associations include: sickle cell disease, HIV, diabetes, heroin, sialidosis, Fabry's disease, and also excess filtering through a limited number of glomeruli due to congenital reductions in glomeruli number (oligonephropathies, renal agenesis, and surgical resection). Unlike minimal change disease, up to 60% of these patients develop end-stage renal disease and are generally steroid unresponsive. Even if a patient receives a kidney transplant, the new kidney also eventually becomes clogged in about 50% of cases.

MEMBRANOUS GLOMERULONEPHRITIS

- Histology: thickened glomerular basement membrane with subepithelial deposits but no proliferative changes
- Aetiology: primary idiopathic and secondary (see associations)
- Pathogenesis: immune-complex deposition
- Associations:
  - cancer of the bowel and bronchus
  - penicillamine, captopril, gold and heavy metals (mercury and cadmium)
  - infections, such as hepatitis B virus, *Schistosoma mansoni*, malaria
  - autoimmune disease, such as SLE, RA; sickle cell anaemia
  - epidemiology: more common in adults, with slight male preponderance
- Presentation:
  - spectrum from asymptomatic proteinuria to nephrotic syndrome
  - chronic renal failure
  - hypertension
  - hyperlipidaemia
- Prognosis:
  - one-third of patients have spontaneous remission
  - one-third remain nephrotic
  - one-third progress to chronic renal failure

MESANGIOCAPILLARY GLOMERULONEPHRITIS/MEMBRANOPROLIFERATIVE GLOMERULONEPHRITIS (RARE IN CHILDREN AGED UNDER 5 YEARS)

	MCGN TYPE I	MCGN TYPE II
Histology	Subendothelial immune deposits of IgG, IgM, IgA, C3, and C4	Dense immune deposit disease with C3 along capillary loops, but no Ig
Aetiology	Primary idiopathic Secondary to endocarditis, SLE,	Primary idiopathic hepatitis C virus, shunt nephritis
Associations	C3 nephritic factor (20%–30%) Hypocomplementaemia with low C3 and C4	C3 nephritic factor (70%) Partial lipodystrophy Normal C4 but low C3
Presentation	Mixed nephritic and nephrotic picture in either type	
Prognosis	Gradual deterioration to end-stage renal failure over 10 years Type II prognosis worse than type I Prognosis worse if crescents found on biopsy or initial presentation with nephrotic syndrome	

MCGN: mesangiocapillary glomerulonephritis; C3: complement 3; C4: complement 4.

(ACUTE) POST-STREPTOCOCCAL GLOMERULONEPHRITIS

- Part of the spectrum of MCGN
- Histology: subepithelial 'humps' on electron microscopy and discontinuous granular deposition of complement (C) 3, IgM, and IgG on immunofluorescence
- Aetiology: follows a nephritogenic streptococcal infection of the throat or skin with a latent period of 7–40 days. This helps to distinguish it from IgA disease which causes renal disease to develop at the same time as an URTI
- Epidemiology: mainly affects children, primarily in nondeveloped countries
- Presentation: 90% of cases are subclinical. The remaining 10% develop an acute nephritic syndrome with haematuria, hypertension, oliguria, and oedema. Rarely (<0.5% of cases), patients develop hypertensive encephalopathy with consequent coma and convulsions. Moderate proteinuria may occur, but overt nephrotic syndrome is rare
- Investigations: elevated antistreptolysin O (ASO) titres, IgM, IgG, cryoglobulinaemia, low C3 (90%), low C4 and C2 (more rarely)
- prognosis: 90% have a full recovery from their acute nephritic illness, but a small percentage (10%) progress to chronic renal failure

Other infections that may give rise to glomerulonephritis

These include:

- *Plasmodium malariae*
- HIV (usually focal segmental glomerulosclerosis)
- hantavirus
- *Schistosoma mansoni* (not *S. japonicum*)
- *Mycobacterium leprae*

Note that diagnosis of rapidly progressive glomerulonephritis is by presentation rather than histology; it requires an active sediment in the urine (i.e. red cell casts) and systemic features, such as oliguria (i.e. a fall in glomerular filtration rate) and hypertension. The histological correlate is often the presence of crescents – a feature of heavy inflammation. It can occur with any glomerulonephritis. It is associated with vasculitides, particularly Wegener's granulomatosis, microscopic polyarteritis, SLE and Henoch–Schönlein purpura, and antiglomerular basement membrane (GBM) disease, which is isolated to the kidneys, especially in nonsmokers. The prognosis varies depending on initial severity and crescent formation, but in general all patients progress to end-stage renal failure. A renal biopsy is imperative unless this is contraindicated, such as in cases of a single functioning kidney, bleeding diathesis and uncontrolled hypertension.

OK, if you encyst

Remember that there are two types of polycystic kidney disease:

1) the childhood type which is usually acquired as an autosomal recessive form and is associated with cysts in the liver
2) the adult type which is acquired as an autosomal dominant condition and is associated with cysts in organs other than the kidney, including the pancreas. It has a 10%–15% association with intracranial berry aneurysms and hence a marked increased risk of subarachnoid haemorrhage

OK. Now let's look at some cases.

Q50

A 41-year-old man presents to casualty with progressive haematuria. He and his partner have just returned from a 2-week trekking holiday in Thailand where they both had a bout of transient gastroenteritis. Just over 1 year ago he had a renal transplant, but he is unclear as to "what had gone wrong" with his kidneys. He is aware, however, that at a recent follow-up appointment, he had no sign of infection and a letter states that his tacrolimus levels were adequate. He has needed a hearing aid since his early twenties and is currently on the waiting list to have a cataract operation. His mother and grandfather were also deaf. He never knew his grandfather as he died before he was born. He works in the Department of Social Services and champions several charities for people with both physical and mental disabilities.

ON EXAMINATION

- Bilateral hearing aids
- Bilateral cataracts and corpuscular pigmentation of right retina
- CVS normal except blood pressure = 175/100 mmHg
- Urine dipstick: blood + + +
  protein +
  no leucocytes/glucose

INVESTIGATIONS

- Haemoglobin = 10.8 g/dl
- White cell count = 7.8 x 10^9/l
- Platelets = 145 x 10^9/l
- Plasma urea = 31 mmol/l
- Plasma creatinine = 560 μmol/l
- Urine microscopy: red cell casts
- Anti-GBM antibody positive

CVS: cardiovascular system; GBM: glomerular basement membrane

a) What renal disease has this man developed in his transplanted kidney?

b) How do you explain his retinal findings?

c) What is the underlying condition?

Renal physicians are a funny lot. Quite why one should develop a fascination with urine (or lack of it) mystifies us. The big problem for renal physicians – and hence for you – is that there is often little to find to aid a diagnosis. Only rarely can you feel a massive kidney, and the answer of polycystic kidney disease is usually obvious by then.

No; to make the right diagnosis, you generally have to depend on the history, particularly family history and drug/toxin exposure, and a few tests, particularly urine microscopy and the presence of autoantibodies.

As always, seek out the abnormalities for which there are limited lists of causes. In this case, the obvious abnormal findings are of corpuscular pigmentation of the right retina, acute renal failure, haematuria, red cell casts, and a positive anti-GBM antibody test.

'Corpuscular pigmentation' is the examiners' way of saying 'retinitis pigmentosa', for which you have already learned a list of causes. As usual, write this down now on scrap paper, then check it against the reminder below:

Retinitis pigmentosa

- Friedreich's ataxia: spinal cord atrophy with degeneration of the spinocerebellar tracts, corticospinal tracts, and dorsal columns; peripheral neuropathies; cardiomyopathy; scoliosis and pes cavus
- Refsum's syndrome: polyneuritis, nerve deafness, cerebellar ataxia, and high cerebrospinal fluid protein concentration
- Laurence–Moon–Biedl syndrome
- Alport's syndrome: hereditary nephritis
- Kearns–Sayre syndrome

Which of these is the cause? Well, it ought to be pretty obvious. Nonetheless, if you really wanted confirmation, you might think of the causes of red cell casts. It ought to appear on the list overleaf.

CAST AWAYS!

There are three sorts of casts that offer some help: red cell, white cell, and fatty.

- Red cell casts mean the kidneys are ravaged – in other words, they have had a major insult that is damaging them, causing both protein and red cell leak. The causes are, therefore, 'generally inflammatory and harmful':

generally	glomerulonephritis*
inflammatory	interstitial nephritis*
and	accelerated hypertension
harmful	haemolytic uraemic syndrome

- Fatty casts are due to nefrotic syndrome, for which there is a limited list of causes (see below)

- Neutrophil (white cell) casts go with nephritis. The causes are those starred* above, and pyelonephritis

The other sorts of cast are pretty useless in making a diagnosis. Hyaline casts are very nonspecific, and broad waxy casts are the hyaline casts of chronic renal failure, which are easily fragmented. Granular casts are similarly nonspecific, and are found in all renal disease regardless of severity or chronicity.

In this case, the lists of causes of red cell casts do not help much. They narrow it down to an interstitial nephritis or glomerulonephritis. At least this helps to confirm Alport's syndrome as the likely cause, with further support from the fact that this seems to be a hereditary problem. Both mother and grandfather were deaf, and the grandfather died at a young age.

Alport's syndrome is a hereditary nephritis characterised by haematuria, progressive renal failure, high-tone sensorineural deafness, and a variety of ocular problems – myopia, early cataracts, and retinitis pigmentosa. Its inheritance is X-linked dominant, so that there is no male-to-male transmission. Affected males pass the disease on to all female offspring, and females generally manifest a less severe form of the disease. Only males develop progressive renal failure, while females have asymptomatic haematuria with no progression to renal failure. Similarly, the ocular and auditory abnormalities are more prevalent in males. The development of renal failure in males has a bimodal age distribution of 15–35 years and 45–60 years. Some 5% of patients who are transplanted for Alport's syndrome develop anti-GBM antibodies after transplantation. AC Alport (1880–1959) was a South African renal physician who practised at St Mary's Hospital in London.

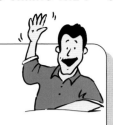

A50

a) **Disease in transplanted kidney**
   Anti-GBM disease has developed

b) **Cause of retinal findings**
   Retinitis pigmentosa

c) **Underlying condition**
   Alport's syndrome

This question may appear in several forms. The examiner may show an audiogram, a retinal photograph showing retinitis pigmentation, a histology slide, or it may even be presented as a 'family tree' with a similar history to the above.

QUIZ SPOT!

UNLUCKY FOR SOME: 13 CAUSES OF PANCYTOPENIA

j	q	b	w	c	e	g	l	e	v	n	b	j	u	t	z	g	a
s	i	b	z	h	j	e	y	z	r	t	a	s	a	s	d	u	l
j	r	v	u	e	r	j	v	m	l	k	l	f	r	e	p	a	r
p	r	i	q	m	x	t	u	b	e	r	c	u	l	o	s	i	s
f	a	n	c	o	n	i	s	o	q	z	o	p	d	k	c	n	b
g	d	a	f	t	l	t	o	f	v	m	h	l	e	f	r	g	d
k	i	s	k	h	z	l	s	r	u	j	o	h	k	a	a	e	l
a	a	g	w	e	o	d	h	t	s	e	l	s	a	k	r	t	u
e	t	u	h	r	t	z	c	e	l	d	y	u	v	e	w	d	r
n	i	r	a	a	v	i	r	a	l	a	j	s	r	u	w	f	o
c	o	d	v	p	m	d	l	s	r	f	l	n	h	t	c	i	u
m	n	w	t	y	l	a	l	l	e	c	u	r	b	r	o	y	h
g	t	I	h	l	w	y	s	s	y	y	i	w	o	k	j	t	s
l	a	t	p	g	v	h	k	s	d	f	h	n	p	g	s	d	q
d	m	v	k	s	u	y	p	l	y	m	p	h	o	m	a	j	d
c	f	g	t	y	l	u	k	j	n	h	s	d	g	m	x	l	r
w	v	o	e	r	t	d	h	g	a	b	d	y	i	o	a	d	t

The answers are on page 256.

Q51

A 35-year-old man is admitted for investigation of leg swelling and abdominal distension, which has developed over the last 6 weeks. He has also felt a little more breathless, but has not noticed any palpitations or experienced any chest pain. About 2 months ago he developed an intensely itchy rash with 'little blisters' on his knees and elbows. He was referred to a dermatologist who gave him a course of medication, which cleared the rash completely. He has had a similar rash in the past though to a lesser degree, which has usually resolved with a slight alteration of his diet. Currently he feels somewhat tired and run-down. He works as a futures trader and has had a stressful few weeks at work. He is good friends with an advertising executive, who has recently been admitted to hospital. Together, they help fund the economies of several small South American countries, *and he can floss his nasal septum*. He denies drinking more than 10 units per week, however, and is a nonsmoker. He lives with his partner of 5 years who also works in the City.

ON EXAMINATION

- Facial, truncal, and limb oedema
- Leuconychia
- No anaemia, cyanosis, clubbing, jaundice, or lymphadenopathy
- Pulse = 96 beats/min
- Blood pressure = 100/55 mmHg
- Jugular venous pressure not elevated
- Heart sounds I + II + S3
- Pitting oedema of lower limbs to trunk
- Respiratory: bibasal dullness to percussion, with reduced air entry and reduced breath sounds on auscultation
- Abdomen: distended but nontender; no palpable organomegaly; shifting dullness, with a fluid thrill

INVESTIGATIONS

- Haemoglobin = 11.8 g/dl
- White cell count = 6.2×10^9/l
- Platelets = 180×10^9/l
- Plasma sodium = 133 mmol/l
- Plasma potassium = 4.0 mmol/l
- Plasma urea = 1.8 mmol/l
- Plasma creatinine = 55 μmol/l
- Serum albumin = 21 g/l
- Serum bilirubin = 15 μmol/l
- Serum alanine aminotransferase = 20 IU/l
- Serum alkaline phosphatase = 105 IU/l
- Plasma glucose = 5.1 mmol/l
- Urinalysis: protein + + +; negative for blood and glucose
- 24-hour urine protein = 4.8 g
- Complement levels (C3 and C4) = Normal

a) What is the cause of this man's presenting complaint?

b) What was the cause of his rash and what treatment did he receive?

c) What is his underlying diagnosis?

d) What is his likely prognosis?

At first glance, there seems little to hang one's hat on. However, the patient has ascites and widespread 'oedema', and a low albumin level. He has heavy proteinuria. Yes! He must have nephrotic syndrome!

Think of your list of causes and jot them down here:

The rash should be identified from the description as being dermatitis herpetiformis. You should remember (from the summary on page 211) that this is associated with Berger's disease. This is also associated with normal complement levels.

A51

a) **Presenting symptoms cause**
   Nephrotic syndrome

b) **Cause of rash; treatment**
   Dermatitis herpetiformis; dapsone

c) **Underlying diagnosis**
   IgA nephropathy or Berger's disease (the commonest primary glomerulonephritis; 80% of cases of nephrotic syndrome arise due to glomerulonephritis)

d) **Prognosis**
   As he has presented with heavy proteinuria, he has a greater than 20% chance of developing end-stage renal failure 20 years post-diagnosis

.... and to finish this renal section.

ANOTHER ODD RENAL LIST: RETROPERITONEAL FIBROSIS

In recent years, this has appeared as a grey case with a characteristic history of dull aching in the abdomen associated with eating and drinking, followed by progressive renal failure, with a diagnostic intravenous pyelogram (IVP), showing medial deviation of the ureters and bilateral hydronephrosis. It can also cause entrapment of the aorta or inferior vena cava, causing arterial insufficiency or venous oedema in the legs.

The causes of this condition include:

- drugs, such as practolol, methysergide
- aortic aneurysm
- lymphoma, radiation
- idiopathic

Treatment is surgical with either stenting of ureters or ureterolysis, which involves dissecting out the ureters carefully from the inflammatory mass, and interpositioning them with a surrounding layer of muscle or peritoneum!

Sex!

The MRCP list of sexual medicine

Sadly, given the pressures of a job and revision, this is probably as close as you're likely to get to the subject. Never mind, it'll be over pretty quickly.

There are few lists to learn and a useful one is for galactorrhoea.

Galactorrhoea

Remember that dopamine is prolactin release inhibitory factor, which is active in the hypothalamic–pituitary axis. Thus, abnormalities in this region can cause galactorrhoea, as can all dopamine-receptor antagonists. The easy ones to remember are:

- pregnancy
- excess oestrogens
- hypothalamic/pituitary lesions
- prolactinoma and ectopic prolactin secretion:
    - bronchogenic carcinoma
    - hypernephroma

Antidopaminergic drugs resulting in elevated prolactin (by virtue of lack of prolactin inhibition):

- phenothiazines
- butyrophenones
- metoclopramide
- methyldopa

The three that are less easy to remember are:

- hypothyroidism
- chronic renal failure
- polycystic ovaries

Other sexy questions usually centre on weird sex-hormone levels. Such cases do not respond well to 'the list approach', but just have to be recognised. We shall therefore run through all the main cases in turn. Just learn to recognise them!

Androgen insensitivity syndrome/testicular feminisation

A defective androgen receptor means that genotypically male children (46XY) have end-organ resistance to testosterone. Some of this excess testosterone is isomerised to oestrogen, so they become phenotypically female. The groin swellings are the undescended testes, the latter being the main risk factor for the development of germ cell tumours of the testes. Therefore, it is usually advised to have bilateral orchidectomy after 21 years of age, but not before this time as the testes are a better source of oestrogens than the oral contraceptive pill.

Congenital adrenal hyperplasia

There are a variety of abnormalities of steroid hormone synthesis that the examiners love to throw in as a quick data question, or even occasionally as an extended grey case. The term 'congenital adrenal hyperplasia' will make many of you groan, but never fear! Below is a simplified scheme of steroid hormone synthesis that is relatively easy to learn and from which you can work out phenotypic appearance and the relevant biochemistry!

Steroid hormone synthesis pathways

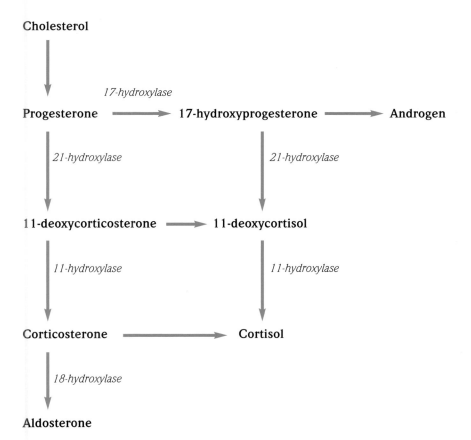

Cholesterol

Progesterone — *17-hydroxylase* → 17-hydroxyprogesterone ——→ Androgen

21-hydroxylase *21-hydroxylase*

11-deoxycorticosterone ——→ 11-deoxycortisol

11-hydroxylase *11-hydroxylase*

Corticosterone ————————→ Cortisol

18-hydroxylase

Aldosterone

Remember this? Keeps cropping up, a bit like the coagulation casacade! Needs to be swotted up for the exam I'm afraid.

KEY FACTS

- For the purposes of understanding the pathways, 11-deoxycorticosterone and 11-deoxycortisol behave like aldosterone and cortisol, respectively.
- All the congenital adrenal hyperplasias are autosomal recessive, with the genes on chromosome 6, so the question may incorporate other siblings!

In terms of sexual precocity, remember the following rules:

- breast development is very sensitive to *oestrogens*, so precocity is usually pituitary
- sexual hair is usually secondary to ambient *testosterone* so precocity is usually adrenal or occasionally ovarian in origin.

Right. That is all you need to know to be able to work out the phenotypes. Practice by filling in the following table:

ENZYME DEFECT	AMBIGUOUS GENITALIA		SALT LOSS	HIGH BP	PUBERTY	ACTH	RENIN
	MALES	FEMALES					
21-hydroxylase	No	Yes	Yes	No	Precocious	High	High
17-hydroxylase							
11-hydroxylase							

ACTH: adrenocorticotrophic hormone; BP: blood pressure.

DIAGNOSTIC INVESTIGATIONS

The diagnostic investigations are as follows:

- 21-hydroxy deficiency: measurement of 17-hydroxyprogesterone and cortisol after tetracosactrin
- 17-hydroxy deficiency: measurement of 11-deoxycorticosterone:cortisol ratio
- 11-hydroxy deficiency: as for 21-hydroxy deficiency

The most common congenital adrenal hyperplasia is 21-hydroxy deficiency (about 95% of cases). However, it is almost invariably a partial deficiency, as complete deficiency presents in the first day of life with a salt-losing crisis.

Q52

A 16-year-old girl is investigated for primary amenorrhoea. At the age of 10 years she began to develop secondary sexual characteristics, but still has not started to menstruate. Both her parents are alive and well. She is an only child. Apart from this she has never needed to see her GP, as she has always been well.

On examination

- Looks well, with well-developed breasts, scanty pubic hair and small bilateral groin swellings
- Pulse = 80 beats/min
- Blood pressure = 110/70 mmHg

Investigations

- Aldosterone = Normal
- Cortisol = Normal
- Testosterone = Elevated
- Oestradiol = Low
- 17-hydroxylase = Normal
- 21-hydroxylase = Normal

a) What is the diagnosis?

b) How would you confirm this?

c) What management steps would you take now and in the future?

The essence of this case is that we have an apparent female with groin swelling and an elevated testosterone level.

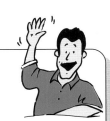

A52

a) Diagnosis
Testicular feminisation

b) Test
Buccal smear or sex chromosome analysis

c) Management
Advise parents to continue raising daughter as female
Counselling may be required
Orchidectomy after the age of 21 years, with exogenous administration of oestrogens

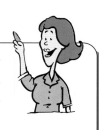

Q53 A 16-year-old girl is being investigated for primary amenorrhoea. She not only has not started menstruating, but also has somewhat under-developed secondary sexual characteristics. She lives with her parents who are alive and well and she is an only child.

ON EXAMINATION

- Fundoscopy reveals scattered flame haemorrhages and exudates
- Pulse = 85 beats/min
- Blood pressure = 170/100 mmHg

INVESTIGATIONS

- ACTH elevated
- Renin undetectable

ACTH: adrenocorticotrophic hormone.

a) What is the diagnosis?

b) How would you confirm this?

This is a case of absent puberty, with low renin levels and hypertension as a result of high ACTH levels.

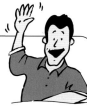

A53
a) **Diagnosis**
   17-hydroxylase deficient congenital adrenal hyperplasia

b) **Test**
   11-deoxycorticosterone level elevated compared to a reduced cortisol level

Q54

A dermatologist sees a 19-year-old girl for acne. She has always had slightly oily skin, but her spots have become much worse in the last year. Further questioning reveals that her menstrual periods have also become more irregular with her cycle varying between 21 and 40 days. She has also noticed an occasional discharge from her breasts. Her 16-year-old sister has normal periods and her mother's cycle has always been regular. Both her parents are well other than that her father takes antiepileptic drugs since he suffered a road traffic accident. The patient has never been in hospital before.

ON EXAMINATION

- Hirsute
- Height = 1.5 m
- Weight = 67 kg
- Marked acne on face and torso
- Galactorrhoea

INVESTIGATIONS

- Oestradiol = 500 (220–1480) pmol/l
- Testosterone = 45 (9–35) nmol/l
- LH = 18 (1–10) IU/l
- FSH = 0.5 (1–7) IU/l
- Prolactin = 800 (70–460) mIU/l
- SHBG = Low

FSH: follicle-stimulating hormone; LH: luteinising hormone; SHBG: sex hormone binding globulin.

a) What is the most likely diagnosis?

b) What other differential diagnosis would you consider?

c) How would you best investigate and treat this girl?

This is a case of absent puberty, with low renin levels and hypertension as a result of high ACTH levels.

- hirsutism
- acne
- obesity
- galactorrhoea
- irregular menstruation
- elevated LH:FSH ratio
- elevated testosterone

There is only one answer – polycystic ovary syndrome. You just have to recognise this, we're afraid. The father's anticonvulsants, which cause hirsutism (phenytoin), have been thrown in as a red herring, but the biochemical abnormalities would not be found in such a case.

Polycystic ovary syndrome diagnosis is primarily clinical, with the biochemistry confirming what one already suspects. In addition to a high testosterone level and LH:FSH ratio (>3), prolactin may also be elevated. This gives rise to the occasional finding in polycystic ovary syndrome of galactorrhoea. Remember that it is only the oestrogen-primed breast that can lactate, which is why men with bronchogenic carcinoma ectopically secreting prolactin do not experience galactorrhoea.

The only possible differential diagnosis would be mild, late-onset 21-hydroxy deficiency congenital adrenal hyperplasia. However, these patients would not experience galactorrhoea for the reasons outlined above.

A54
a) **Diagnosis**
Polycystic ovary syndrome

b) **Possible differential diagnosis**
Mild, late-onset 21-hydroxy deficiency congenital adrenal hyperplasia

c) **Investigations and treatment**
Ultrasound scan of ovaries to reveal multiple (>5), small (<1 cm) cysts. Treat with monthly progestogen

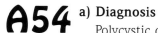

11
MOPPING UP

My first MRCP book

This section is designed to provide you with 'cannon fodder' for practice. It should allow you to practice using your lists. We will also try to cover a few more of the 'just recognise it' classic cases, and any of the other 'general bits and bobs' we have so far missed out. Once you have done all of these, we suggest that you quickly run through all the lists once more to make sure that you know them all. We have printed them all at the back of the book for you to remove, so that you can carry them with you as an *aide-mémoire*. We strongly recommend that you now get hold of a selection of the other 'MRCP books' on the shelves, and use their questions for practice.

The MRCP examination is not easy, and can be a bit demoralising. However, the strategies you learn *will* be useful to you in the future: there really is no better doctor than the general medical registrar who has just passed the MRCP examination. Certainly our choice of doctors when we get poorly.

Good luck!

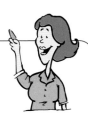

Q55

A 45-year-old woman presents with breathlessness and lethargy. She has a past history of treated hypertension. On examination she appears anaemic and her chest is clear.

INVESTIGATIONS	RESULTS
Haemoglobin	7.6 g/dl
White cell count	3.6 x 10^9/l
Platelets	235 x 10^9/l
Plasma sodium	134 mmol/l
Plasma potassium	4.6 mmol/l
Plasma urea	6.7 mmol/l
Plasma creatinine	65 μmol/l
Serum bilirubin	28 μmol/l
Serum aspartate aminotransferase	12 IU/l
Serum alanine aminotransferase	9 IU/l
Serum alkaline phosphatase	121 IU/l
Reticulocyte count	11%
Chest X-ray	Slight cardiomegaly
Electrocardiogram	Voltage criteria for LVH

LVH: left ventricular hypertrophy.

a) What is the diagnosis of her recent problem?

b) What would you expect to find in the urine?

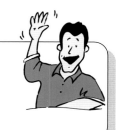

A55   **a) Diagnosis**
Methyldopa-induced haemolytic anaemia

b) Urine test
Raised urinary urobilinogen, haemosiderinuria

This question should have been easy for you by now. The only problem is to discover the cause of her haemolysis. As we have previously stated in this book, think of the drugs. In this case, the patient has been treated long-term with methyldopa. It sounds as though it is time for a change. Bring her hypertension treatment up to date.

Remember the classic laboratory features associated with haemolytic anaemia:

- raised serum unconjugated bilirubin
- raised methaemoglobulinaemia
- raised urinary urobilinogen
- raised faecal stercobilinogen
- haemosiderinuria
- absent serum haptoglobins

ANSWERS TO PRESENTATION PUZZLE (see page 144)

Here are the diseases, and presenting features:

	Disease			
	Carpal Tunnel	**BHL**	**Bronchiectasis**	**Lung Fibrosis**
George	Acromegaly	Sarcoid	Kartagener's	Sarcoid
Michael	TB	TB	TB	TB
Sarah	Pregnancy	TB	TB	Pigeons
Nicky	TB	Phenytoin	Aspergillus	TB
Peter	Gout	CF	CF	Amiodarone
Ruth	RA	EAA	Yellow Nail	EAA

George and Ruth are the least infected. Neither has an infectious disease. Peter has cystic fibrosis, and thus chronic chest infection. Serum ACE might be elevated in all the patients. Although sarcoid classically raises serum ACE, so too does lung fibrosis in general. This is perhaps especially true of tuberculous scarring.

Q56

An 82-year-old man presents with general lethargy and weakness. He was reasonably well until 3 months ago, although he has suffered with nose bleeds for the last 4 years. His brother who lives with him has been treated for hypertension with nifedipine for many years. Two months ago the patient also had an episode of coughing up clotted blood and has felt short of breath since then, although he has had a good exercise tolerance. There is no significant past medical history except for an episode of typhoid fever whilst in the Army in North Africa in 1942. He smokes five cigarettes per day. On examination he is pale and appears short of breath with dry skin and mucous membranes.

INVESTIGATIONS	RESULTS
Haemoglobin	9.9 g/dl
White cell count	12.6 x 10⁹/l
Platelets	123 x 10⁹/l
Plasma sodium	131 mmol/l
Plasma potassium	6.7 mmol/l
Plasma urea	32 mmol/l
Plasma creatinine	290 μmol/l
Serum bilirubin	9 μmol/l
Serum aspartate aminotransferase	9 IU/l
Serum alanine aminotransferase	18 IU/l
Serum alkaline phosphatase	65 IU/l
Hepatitis B serum antigen	Negative
Serum creatinine kinase	120 IU/l
Urinalysis	Red cell casts
Chest X-ray	Cavitating lesions in left upper zone and right lower zone
Antiglomerular basement membrane (GBM)	Negative
Antinuclear antibodies	Negative
Antidouble-stranded DNA	Negative
Rhesus factor	Negative

a) What is the most likely diagnosis?

b) Give three tests to confirm the diagnosis

This question requires you to put together a number of your well-known lists; in particular, the causes of lung cavitation and the causes of renal failure with red cell casts in the urine. Cover the page and write these down now.

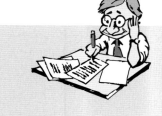

CAUSES OF CAVITATION ON A CHEST X-RAY

Cancers cause cavities, so can TB
Wegener's, rheumatoid†, also PE.
Think of the 'oses' of which there are three
Also of abscesses, Klebsielli.*

The three 'oses': histoplasmosis, coccidioidomycosis, and aspergillosis

Abscesses: think staphylococci, Klebsiella, amoebiasis, aspiration

* small cell lung cancer
† and progressive massive fibrosis/rheumatoid nodules associated with rheumatoid arthritis (RA)
  TB: tuberculosis; Wegener's: Wegener's granulomatosis; PE: pulmonary embolism

CAUSES OF RENAL FAILURE

- Harmful   Haemolytic uraemic syndrome
- And   Accelerated hypertension
- Inflammatory Interstitial nephritis
- Generally   Glomerulonephritis

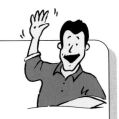

A56   **a) Diagnosis**
Wegener's granulomatosis

b) Tests
Nasal biopsy
Renal biopsy
Antineutrophil cytoplasmic antibodies (ANCA)
Transbronchial biopsy
Open lung biopsy

Cavitation plus casts really only leaves Wegener's granulomatosis. The presence of nasal symptoms (caused by nasal granuloma) clinches it. Always go for the least invasive site for biopsy.

At this point we will briefly discuss the various merits of the ANCA tests.

ANCA

There are two main types of ANCA test: C-ANCA and P-ANCA

- Cytoplasmic antineutrophil cytoplasmic antibodies (C-ANCA) stain the cytoplasm diffusely; these antibodies are usually directed against a serine protease called proteinase 3 (PR3).
- Perinuclear antineutrophil cytoplasmic antibodies (P-ANCA) are usually directed against myeloperoxidase (MPO).

For C-ANCA-positive vasculitis, the level of C-ANCA, C-reactive protein, and renal function can be used to assess disease activity. As in antiglomerular basement membrane (GBM) disease, if there is pulmonary involvement, transfer coefficients (KCOs) can be used as a marker of the degree of pulmonary vasculitis.

Most importantly, for P-ANCA vasculitis you *cannot* use titre to monitor disease activity.

A small number of patients may be both C-ANCA and anti-GBM antibody-positive, and these patients have a particularly poor prognosis.

ASSOCIATIONS

C-ANCA: Wegener's granulomatosis (WG, positive in 95% of patients).
(C-ANCA = W-ANCA; i.e. C-ANCA is positive in WG.)

P-ANCA: unlike C-ANCA, this is a bit promiscuous and is found in many diseases, including:

- microscopic polyarteritis
- polyarteritis nodosa
- and a variety of rheumatic autoimmune diseases, including:
  - RA
  - systemic lupus erythematosus (SLE)
  - Sjögren's syndrome
  - polymyositis
  - dermatomyositis

If P-ANCA is directed against MPO, then it is relatively specific to (though not sensitive for) microscopic polyarteritis and polyarteritis nodosa.

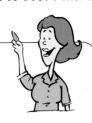

Q57

A 43-year-old woman originally resident in Hong Kong presents with progressive lethargy for the last year. In addition she has lost 2 stone in weight, felt nauseous, and has been anorexic. Her husband has also noted that her eyes have appeared yellow on a number of occasions.

INVESTIGATIONS	RESULTS
Haemaglobin	11.8 g/dl
White cell count	6.3 x 10⁹/l
Platelets	190 x 10⁹/l
ESR	42 mm in first hour
Plasma sodium	130 mmol/l
Plasma potassium	3.9 mmol/l
Plasma urea	6.9 mmol/l
Serum bilirubin	37 (3–17) μmol/l
Serum alanine aminotransferase	63 (5–15) IU/l
Serum alkaline phosphatase	83 (0–95) IU/l
Clotting INR	1.1
Thrombin time	Normal
Serum IgG	24 g/l
Serum IgM	5.3 g/l
Serum IgA	2.5 g/l

ESR: erythrocyte sedimentation rate; INR: international normalised ratio. Figures in parentheses indicate normal ranges.

a) What is the most likely diagnosis?

b) What three investigations would you do next?

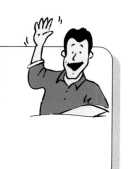

A57 a) **Diagnosis**
Chronic active hepatitis

b) **Investigations**
Liver biopsy
Hepatitis serology (hepatitis B, C, D)
Antinuclear antibody

We didn't think this question needed a lot of explanation. We are sure that by now you will be getting these right!!

Quiz Spot!

Jigsaw Puzzle: Retinitis Pigmentosa and Angioid Retinal Streaks

Fit the following jigsaw pieces into the grid to reveal causes of retinitis pigmentosa and of angioid retinal streaks. Just to make life tricky, there is one box missing. What are the diseases, and which causes which eye sign? The answers are on page 270.

Q58

A 58-year-old man presents to casualty with right-sided visual loss. He is a nonsmoker, with no previous history of ischaemic heart disease or hypercholesterolaemia. He drinks about 27 units of alcohol per week, though this may be more during weeks when he is entertaining clients. He has occasionally taken cocaine. He works in the advertising industry and has recently been headhunted to be an executive for a large, London-based firm. At that time, a medical examination was said to show a 'muscular heart' on electrocardiogram (ECG). On systems review, he admits to having an approximately 2-month history of intermittent left-sided loin pain and fevers and he thinks he has lost some weight. His GP recently started him on atenolol treatment in a well-man clinic.

On examination

- He appears flushed, but has no lymphadenopathy, jaundice, cyanosis, clubbing, or oedema
- Blood pressure = 178/100 mm Hg
- Pulse = 88 beats/min
- Temperature = 38.2°C
- Cardiovascular examination otherwise normal
- Respiratory examination otherwise normal
- Abdominal examination is unremarkable except for a left varicocoele
- Right homonymous hemianopia, with no other neurological deficit

Investigations

- Haemoglobin = 19.2 g/dl
- White cell count = 8.2 x 10^9/l
- Platelets = 420 x 10^9/l
- ESR = 58 mm in first hour
- Plasma sodium = 138 mmol/l
- Plasma potassium = 4.5 mmol/l
- Plasma creatinine = 159 μmol/l
- Plasma urea = 7.8 mmol/l
- Urinalysis: protein + +, blood + + +
- Urine 24-hour VMA elevated

ESR: erythrocyte sedimentation rate; VMA: vanillylmandelic acid.

a) What is the haematological diagnosis?

b) What is the cause of this patient's presenting complaint?

c) How do you explain the left varicocoele?

d) What is the underlying diagnosis?

Well. What do we know? This coke-head has some systemic illness (weight loss, fever, elevated ESR), neurological signs (right homonymous hemianopia), polycythaemia (haemoglobin 19.2 g/dl) and renal pathology (haematuria, proteinuria, left varicocoele). He also has an elevated urinary VMA.

Let's start with what you know already. Revise the causes of polycythaemia.

CAUSES OF POLYCYTHAEMIA

- Relative: dehydration, Gaisböck's syndrome (stress)
- Primary: polycythaemia rubra vera (PRV) (splenomegaly, raised platelets)
- Secondary: hypoxia, chronic obstructive pulmonary disease (COPD), altitude abnormal haemoglobin, sleep apnoea
- Excess erythropoietin: cerebellar haemangioma, hepatoma, phaechromocytoma, hypernephroma, polycystic/transplant kidneys, uterine leiomyomata/fibromata

Now exclude the unlikely ones by scoring through them with a pen.
Hopefully, the list will be a lot smaller (and won't contain uterine fibromata!):

- Primary: PRV
- Secondary: hypoxia
- Excess erythropoietin: cerebellar haemangioma, hepatoma, hypernephroma

This patient has several systemic features suggestive of an underlying malignancy. The reported neurology does not fit with a cerebellar haemangioma. Hepatoma or hypernephroma seem the best choices. Which is the best fit? The varicocoele is explicable on the basis that tumour invasion of the left renal vein is interfering with the drainage of the left testicular vein (the right testicular vein drains directly into the inferior vena cava).

Therefore, go with the diagnosis of hypernephroma… and you'd be right!!!

The elevated VMA result is thrown in as a red herring; false positive VMA results can be seen in hypernephromas.

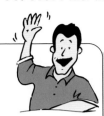

A58
a) **Haematological diagnosis**
Secondary polycythaemia

b) **Cause of presenting complaint**
Right occipital thromboembolic infarct

c) **Cause of varicocoele**
Impaired drainage of left testicular vein due to tumour invasion of left renal vein

d) **Underlying diagnosis**
Left renal cell carcinoma (hypernephroma)

HYPERNEPHROMA

Hypernephroma may be presented as a question in different ways.

- pyrexia of unknown origin: renal cell carcinoma (RCC) is the classic oncological cause

- hypercalcaemia: in addition to secreting erythropoietin, RCC may secrete parathyroid hormone-related peptide (PTHrP). As a result of hypercalcaemia, the patient in the case history may present with polydipsia and polyuria

- musculoskeletal: paraneoplastic syndromes of RCC are classically musculoskeletal, and patients may present with vasculitis, giant cell arteritis, myositis, or polymyalgia

Q59

A 75-year-old man who is under treatment for prostatic carcinoma presents with lethargy and weakness. He has been taking cyproterone acetate for the last 4 years and his prostate-specific antigen (PSA) level was less than 10 ng/ml when checked 6 months ago. Over the last 3 weeks he has been breathless, with reduced exercise tolerance. He used to be able to walk his dog 3 miles, but can now only walk about half a mile. He has been a smoker for the last 60 years having started at school, but only smokes 3 cigarettes per day. He drinks 2 pints of beer per day. He does not have a cough and has not had any haemoptysis. On examination he is pale, his chest is clinically clear, and cardiovascular examination is unremarkable.

INVESTIGATIONS	RESULTS
Haemoglobin	$7.3 \times 10^9/l$
Mean corpuscular volume	83 fl
Platelets	$203 \times 10^9/l$
Plasma sodium	135 mmol/l
Plasma potassium	4.5 mmol/l
Plasma urea	4.3 mmol/l
Plasma creatinine	76 μmol/l
Serum bilirubin	8 μmol/l
Serum aspartate aminotransferase	12 IU/l
Serum alanine aminotransferase	9 IU/l
Serum alkaline phosphatase	98 IU/l
Chest X-ray	Normal
FEV_1	3.2 l
FVC	3.8 l
Blood film	Multiple fragmented red cells and burr cells

FEV_1: forced expiratory volume in 1 second; FVC: forced vital capacity.

a) What is the diagnosis?

Again, this question may appear difficult on the surface, with multiple possible causes of his shortness of breath. The anaemia is clearly pathological and could be caused by a number of factors, including bone marrow carcinomatous infiltration, drug-induced direct suppression, and intestinal bleeding. However, the blood film gives the answer away. As discussed previously, in the MRCP examination there are classic questions and classic associations. In this case, the fragmented red cells and burr cells should immediately alert you to the problem of microangiopathic haemolytic anaemia (MAHA). All it then requires is for you to identify the cause from all the rubbishy information that you have been given. Of importance is the fact that he is being treated for prostatic cancer, and although this has been well controlled, it must be the cause of his problem.

A59 a) Diagnosis
MAHA secondary to prostatic cancer

Remind yourselves of the causes of this condition. Write them in the space below, then look at the list that follows.

CAUSES OF MICROANGIOPATHIC HAEMOLYTIC ANAEMIA (MAHA)

- growths: cancers; foetuses (eclampsia, abruption, intrauterine death, amniotic fluid embolus)
- damage to small vessels: malignant hypertension, vasculitides, burns, sepsis, and disseminated intravascular coagulation (DIC)
- renal failure-associated: thrombotic thrombocytopenic purpura (TTP); haemolytic uraemic syndrome (HUS); acute glomerulonephritis
- drugs: such as cytotoxic agents, cyclosporin

Q60 A 26-year-old man was seen in the fertility clinic with his wife. He complained of low libido and was concerned at his lack of sexual development. He claimed to shave only once every 1–2 weeks. Otherwise he had no significant past medical history and has only occasionally used arnica for chilblains.

ON EXAMINATION

- Height = 1.96 m
- Weight = 75 kg
- Bilateral gynaecomastia
- Scanty pubic hair
- Small testes

INVESTIGATIONS

- Serum testosterone = 7 (9–35) nmol/l
- Serum LH = 16 (1–10) IU/l
- Serum FSH = 28 (1–7) IU/l
- Serum HCG = <5 IU/l

FSH: follicle-stimulating hormone; HCG: human chorionic gonadotrophin; LH: luteinising hormone. Figures in parentheses represent normal ranges.

a) What is the underlying diagnosis?

b) How would you confirm this?

Hypogonadism plus gynaecomastia plus tall and slim!

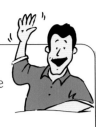

A60 **a) Diagnosis**
Primary hypogonadism secondary to Klinefelter's syndrome

b) Test
Chromosomal analysis (47XXY)

FEATURES OF KLINEFELTER'S SYNDROME

- Tall
- Gynaecomastia
- Usually of normal intelligence
- Azoospermia with small testes

- Diabetes mellitus
- Autoimmune disorders are more common
- Increased risk of breast cancer and leukaemia

Q61 a) What is the type of inheritance shown?

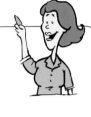

b) Name five conditions inherited in this manner.

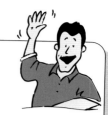

A61

a) Inheritance type
Sex-linked recessive

b) Sex-linked recessive conditions inherited
Duchenne muscular dystrophy
Becker-type muscular dystrophy
Chronic granulomatous disease
Glucose-6-phosphate dehydrogenase deficiency
Haemophilia A
Haemophilia B
Fabry's disease
Alport's syndrome

That came a bit out of the blue didn't it? We apologise wholeheartedly for including a genetic diagram such as this. The only problem is that this type of question has come up in the past. Just remember the patterns. We hope this type of question can be eliminated in the future. (If you are a keen geneticist then we wish you all the best for an exciting career. No, honestly!!)

QUIZ SPOT!

Q: Who were the three 'born unlucky' as causes of peripheral neuropathy?
And who were the three dejected, two infected, two injected, one connected, and the granulomata suspected as causes?

A: See page 42.

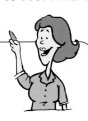

Q62

A 13-year-old girl is seen in casualty with sudden onset of shortness of breath that occurred in a lesson at school. On arrival in casualty, an arterial blood gas is taken on air.

INVESTIGATIONS	RESULTS
pH	7.63
pCO_2	2.6 kPa
pO_2	17.8 kPa
Bicarbonate	22 mmol/l
Chest X-ray	Normal
ECG	Normal

a) What is the most likely diagnosis?

b) What diagnosis must be excluded?

c) How would you manage this girl?

This patient has respiratory alkalosis.

CAUSES OF RESPIRATORY ALKALOSIS

- pneumonia
- pulmonary embolism
- pneumothorax
- early stages of salicylate overdose
- hysterical hyperventilation

Most are unlikely on the basis of the other investigations. This makes hysterical hyperventilation the most likely. As a point of examination technique, the examiners do not like you putting paper bags over patient's faces, so reassurance is therefore the correct answer to part c.

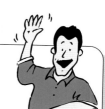

A62 **a) Diagnosis**
Respiratory alkalosis secondary to hyperventilation

b) Exclude
Pulmonary embolus (salicylate overdose in its early stages)

c) Management
Reassurance

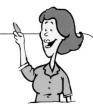

Q63

A 27-year-old homosexual man returns from a visit to India. Prior to his visit he had been well except for one episode of nonspecific urethritis that was treated at a sexually transmitted disease (STD) clinic 3 years ago. This settled the symptoms and he has had no further STDs. Before travelling to India, he contacted his local travel clinic and was vaccinated for hepatitis A, hepatitis B, typhoid, and cholera. Furthermore, he took antimalarial drugs as prescribed. During the visit, he was careful about hygiene and only ate in hotels, drank bottled water, and swam in the hotel pool. Two days after his return, he developed a febrile illness, associated with a diffuse rash and a sore throat. He went to see his GP, who noticed that in addition to the maculo-papular rash he had diffuse lymphadenopathy and a smooth, 1 cm enlargement of the liver. His throat was reddened with a white exudate. In addition, he was febrile with a temperature of 37.4°C.

INVESTIGATIONS	RESULTS
3 x malarial screens	Negative
Haemoglobin	12.3 g/dl
White cell count	12.5 x 10⁹/l
Lymphocytes	90%
Platelets	140 x 10⁹/l
Urinalysis and electrolytes	Normal
Monospot	Negative
CMV	Negative
TPHA	Negative
FTA-ABS	Negative
HIV I/II	Negative
Antistreptolysin O titre	Negative
Chest X-ray	NAD
Blood culture	Negative
Urine culture	Negative
Throat culture	Negative

CMV: cytomegalovirus; FTA-ABS: fluorescent treponemal antibody absorbed test; NAD: no abnormality detected; TPHA: *Treponema pallidum* haemagglutination

a) What is the most likely diagnosis?

b) What test would you perform to confirm your diagnosis?

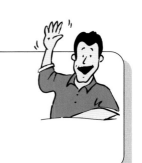

A63 a) **Diagnosis**
HIV seroconversion illness

b) **Test**
P24 Ag test
Repeat HIV test in 3 months

This is one of the classic MRCP examination questions and this type of question is difficult to cover easily in a text of this size. You are faced with a patient who has been abroad and who, to all intents and purposes, has glandular fever, and yet every test that you are given is negative. This should therefore alert you to the fact that this is a 'catch-question'. If you work through the possible causes of a glandular fever-like illness – CMV, Epstein–Barr virus (EBV), or HIV – then there really isn't any problem. You are left with only one possible diagnosis, so treat yourself and write it down!

We are sorry that we couldn't cover how to answer this question within the book before now. But now you have seen it!

SOLUTION TO SIADH CIRCLE (see page 178)

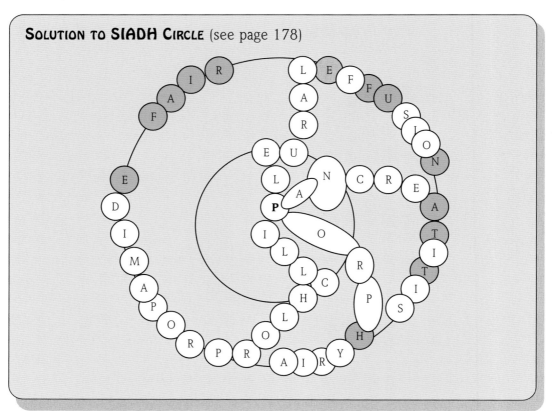

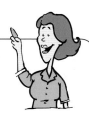

Q64

A 53-year-old man presents to the respiratory outpatient clinic with increasing shortness of breath. He has never smoked. His lung function tests are recorded below.

Test	Patient	Predicted
FEV$_1$	2.2 l	4.5 l
FVC	2.8 l	5.2 l
TLC	4.5 l	6.0 l
DLCO	14 ml/min/mmHg	24 ml/min/mmHg

DLCO: diffusing capacity for carbon monoxide; FEV$_1$: forced expiratory volume in 1 second ; FVC: forced vital capacity; TLC: total lung capacity.

a) What does this test reveal?

b) What is the most likely diagnosis?

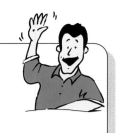

A64 a) **Test reveals**
   A restrictive lung defect

   b) **Diagnosis**
   Cryptogenic fibrosing alveolitis

A number of classic patterns of pulmonary function appear in the MRCP examination. To understand these requires knowledge of the meaning of the various types of lung volume.

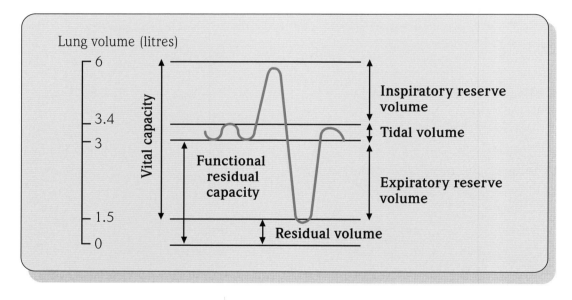

A restrictive pattern results in the reduction in both FEV_1 and FVC with a normal FEV_1/FVC ratio. These diseases result in a significant reduction in TLC with parallel reduction in the functional residual capacity, residual volume (RV), and vital capacity. Furthermore, there is a reduction in the carbon monoxide transfer factor, TLCO (or KCO [transfer coefficient of carbon monoxide] when TLCO is corrected for lung volumes), due to inefficiency of the lungs.

Causes of a low **TLCO**

- Emphysema
- Pulmonary emboli
- Pulmonary fibrosis
- Ageing
- Pulmonary oedema
- Low cardiac output states

Causes of a raised **TLCO**

- Asthma (although TLCO can also be normal)
- Pulmonary haemorrhage (Wegener's granulomatosis, Goodpasture's syndrome)
- Left-to-right cardiac shunting

An obstructive pulmonary function test pattern results in a reduction in peak expiratory flow rate and FEV_1 with a reduction in the FEV_1/FVC ratio. Typically, the FVC is normal in early disease, but is reduced in more severe disease as the RV is increased as a consequence of air trapping.

Liver line-up answers (see page 101)

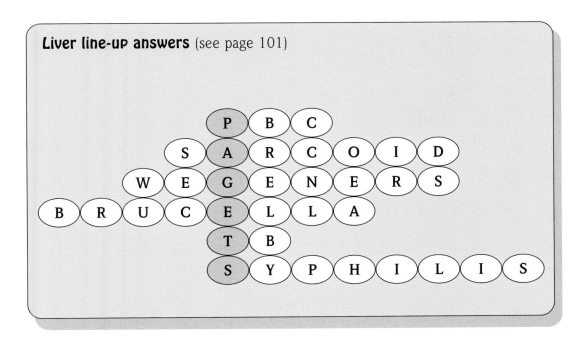

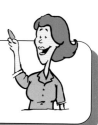

Q65

A 36-year-old man, had a cardiac catheterisation as part of his investigation for breathlessness. The following data were obtained.

CAVITY	PRESSURE (MMHG)
Right atrial end - diastolic	8
Right ventricular end - diastolic	4
Pulmonary wedge	19
Pulmonary artery	64/32
Left ventricular end - diastolic	12

a) What are the most likely valve abnormalities?

UNLUCKY FOR SOME ANSWERS (see page 219):

alcohol, brucella, carcinoma, chemotherapy, drugs, Fanconi's, irradiation, lymphoma, PNH, SLE, thymic tumours, tuberculosis, viral

j	q	b	w	c	e	g	l	e	v	n	b	j	u	t	z	g	a
s	i	b	z	h	j	e	y	z	r	t	a	s	a	s	d	u	l
j	r	v	u	e	r	j	v	m	l	k	l	f	r	e	p	a	r
p	r	i	q	m	x	t	u	b	e	r	c	u	l	o	s	i	s
f	a	n	c	o	n	i	s	o	q	z	o	p	d	k	c	n	b
g	d	a	f	t	l	t	o	f	v	m	h	l	e	f	r	g	d
k	i	s	k	h	z	l	s	r	u	j	o	h	k	a	a	e	l
a	a	g	w	e	o	d	h	t	s	e	l	s	a	k	r	t	u
e	t	u	h	r	t	z	c	e	l	d	y	u	v	e	w	d	r
n	i	r	a	a	v	i	r	a	l	a	j	s	r	u	w	f	o
c	o	d	v	p	m	d	l	s	r	f	l	n	h	t	c	i	u
m	n	w	t	y	l	a	l	l	e	c	u	r	b	r	o	y	h
g	t	l	h	l	w	y	s	s	y	y	i	w	o	k	j	t	s
l	a	t	p	g	v	h	k	s	d	f	h	n	p	g	s	d	q
d	m	v	k	s	u	y	p	l	y	m	p	h	o	m	a	j	d
c	f	g	t	y	l	u	k	j	n	h	s	d	g	m	x	l	r
w	v	o	e	r	t	d	h	g	a	b	d	y	i	o	a	d	t

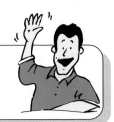

A65 a) Likely abnormalities
Tricuspid stenosis and mitral stenosis

MEAN (RANGE) NORMAL CARDIAC PRESSURES (MMHG)

Right atrial	Mean	4 (0–8)
Right ventricular	Systolic	25 (15–30)
	Diastolic	4 (0–8)
Pulmonary artery	Systolic	25 (15–30)
	Diastolic	10 (5–15)
	Mean	15 (10–20)
Left atrial	Mean	7 (4–12)
Left ventricular	Systolic	120 (90–140)
	Diastolic	7 (4–12)
Aortic	Systolic	120 (90–140)
	Diastolic	70 (60–90)
	Mean	85 (70–105)

QUIZ SPOT!

Q: What are the causes of cerebrospinal fluid lymphocytosis?

A: See page 41 for our list.

Q66

A 32-year-old man presents to casualty with a decreased level of consciousness. He was well until 3 hours previously when he complained of feeling cold. He was driven away from work by a friend, but seemed increasingly lethargic, became confused, and then rapidly lost consciousness. Previously he has been relatively fit except for an episode of pneumonia as a child. He is not receiving any medication, drinks only a moderate amount alcohol, and smokes 10 cigarettes per day.

INVESTIGATIONS	RESULTS
Temperature	38.5°C
Blood pressure	90/50 mm Hg
Pulse	110 beats/min
Kernig's sign	Negative
Meningism	Negative
Glasgow Coma Scale	8
Lower limbs	Diffuse nonblanching petechial rash

a) **What is the most likely diagnosis?**

b) **What is the first thing that you would do?**

c) **Give two tests to confirm your diagnosis.**

A66

a) **Diagnosis**
   Meningococcal septicaemia

b) **Management**
   Give high-dose intravenous benzylpenicillin (or ceftriaxone)

c) **Tests**
   Blood cultures
   Lumbar puncture (post-CT [computerised tomography] scan if available)
   Meningococcal serology/polymerase chain reaction (PCR)

This question has graced the pages of the MRCP written examination on many occasions. Clearly, most candidates will get it right. However, it is very important that you are precise in your answers. For example meningococcal meningitis would score significantly fewer marks than septicaemia. In part b, most people write penicillin, and this exemplifies the importance of being accurate in your answers.

The issue of serology and PCR is important. In the past, physicians have erroneously held off antibiotics (especially in those with meningitis) in the hope of sending cerebral spinal fluid (CSF)/blood to the laboratory for culture first. Always treat first; you can send off CSF or blood for meningococcal antigen testing many hours after the event.

Always watch out for other complications – your examiners will. Apart from shock, these patients almost all get a coagulopathy, whether or not this is frank disseminated intravascular coagulation (DIC). Remember to correct this; there is evidence that provision of protein C (an anticlotting factor) may improve prognosis, especially in children. This form of meningitis can be complicated by acute haemorrhagic adrenal failure and is known as the Waterhouse–Friderichsen syndrome. In meningitis and in proven septicaemia, remember to treat contacts with rifampicin or ciprofloxacin – Carter got his residency in ER for remembering that!

FOR THE RECORD

Rupert Waterhouse (1872–1958): an English physician

Carl Friderichsen (born 1886): a Danish paediatrician

Q67

A 34-year-old man presents with a deep venous thrombosis of his right leg. He had a similar episode affecting his left leg 3 years ago for which he received warfarin for 3 months with no complications. At the age of 31 years, he presented with an acutely painful eye, which was diagnosed as an anterior uveitis. In addition, he has suffered from recurrent episodes of knee and arm pain and has been investigated by rheumatologists for this, but no diagnosis has been made. He also admits to suffering from mouth ulcers for which he takes over-the-counter remedies.

INVESTIGATIONS	RESULTS
Haemoglobin	12.4 g/dl
White cell count	6.8 (normal differential) x 10⁹/l
Platelets	253 x 10⁹/l
ESR	25 mm in first hour
Plasma sodium	134 mmol/l
Plasma potassium	4.2 mmol/l
Plasma urea	4 mmol/l
Plasma creatinine	89 μmol/l
Liver function tests	Normal
Urinalysis	NAD
Chest X-ray	Normal
Doppler ultrasound right leg	Extensive DVT
ANCA	Negative
Antinuclear antibodies	Negative
Anti-double-stranded DNA	Negative
Rhesus factor	Negative
Ham's acid lysis/acidified serum test	Negative

ANCA: antineutrophil cytoplasmic antibodies; DVT: deep venous thrombosis; ESR: erythrocyte sedimentation rate; NAD: no abnormality detected.

a) **What is the most likely diagnosis?**

b) **How would you confirm the diagnosis?**

c) **What is the inheritance pattern?**

This requires knowledge of a number of lists: the causes of recurrent oral ulceration, anterior uveitis, recurrent deep venous thrombosis, and polyarthropathy (write this last list down or cheat and look it up in the list of lists at the end of the book).

CAUSES OF RECURRENT ORAL ULCERATION

- aphthous ulcers
- inflammatory bowel disease (IBD) (ulcerative colitis/Crohn's disease)*
- Behçet's syndrome*
- Reiter's syndrome*
- seronegative arthritis
- coeliac disease
- other causes of malabsorption (see earlier list, page 153)
- pemphigus (and rarely pemphigoid)
- SLE

*These cause both oral and genital ulcers.

CAUSES OF AN ANTERIOR UVEITIS

- infectious: CMV, toxoplasmosis, syphilis, TB
- neoplastic conditions: lymphomas
- systemic diseases: ankylosing spondylitis, Reiter's syndrome, Behçet's syndrome, sarcoidosis, IBD, psoriatic arthropathy, juvenile arthritis, Kawasaki's disease
- others: drug-induced (e.g. rifabutin)

CAUSES OF RECURRENT DEEP VENOUS THROMBOSIS

- thrombophilia: antithrombin III deficiency, protein S or protein C deficiency, factor V Leiden mutation
- dysfibrinogenaemia
- factor XII deficiency
- malignancy
- surgery and trauma
- postoperative
- drugs: oral contraceptive pill
- hyperhomocystinaemia
- Behçet's syndrome
- antiphospholipid syndrome
- paroxysmal nocturnal haemoglobinuria (see 'A bloody hell', pages 184 and 194)
- nephrotic syndrome

CAUSES OF POLYARTHROPATHY (WHICH YOU KNOW)

If you can remember the first two lists, have a working knowledge of the third, and know the fourth then this question is an absolute gift. However, the final two answers are very difficult and are in fact well above the scope of the MRCP examination. We have put them in to make sure that any smart Alec who has not got a question wrong so far has now!!!

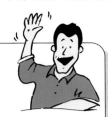

A67

a) **Diagnosis**
   Behçet's syndrome

b) **Test**
   Clinical grounds only! There are no specific tests for
   Behçet's syndrome

c) **Inheritance pattern**
   Unknown. A genetic basis has been suggested, with an increased
   prevalence of histocompatibility class human leucocyte antigen (HLA)-B5.
   Affected children of patients with Behçet's syndrome may have an earlier
   age of onset, which is termed genetic anticipation. In many genetic
   disorders, this characteristic has been linked to an increased number of
   nucleotide repeats within each successive generation

CLINICAL FEATURES OF BEHÇET'S SYNDROME

- Predominantly affects males – HLA-B5

- Predominates along the old trade routes – Japan, China, Iran, Turkey, and
  the Mediterranean

- Oral ulceration

- Genital ulceration (nasty!!)

- Skin: pustules (at venepuncture sites ++), papules, erythema nodosum

- Eye: anterior/posterior uveitis/cataracts

- Neurological disease: aseptic meningitis, cranial nerve palsies

- Vascular: recurrent venous and arterial thromboses

- Arthritis

- Renal disease: usually mild proteinuria; can get amyloidosis

- Gastrointestinal: ulceration

- Treatment: topical or systemic steroids with or without colchicine;
  treat neurological/ocular symptoms with immunosuppressants

Behçet's syndrome is a favourite MRCP examination question and is often a mimic of
arthritides, other autoimmune syndromes, such as SLE/IBD, multiple sclerosis, or more
commonly *Reiter's syndrome.*

The single major difference between Behçet's syndrome and Reiter's syndrome is that the latter
may be caught in the context of pleasure while sufferers of the former have no such luck. More
conventionally, Reiter's syndrome is chronologically related to infections, has different skin and
genito-urinary manifestations (no erythema nodosum or pathergy, but balanitis is present), has
different HLA associations, and less in the way of systemic side-effects.

Q68

A 34-year-old man is admitted to the casualty department with central chest pain of 2 hours duration. The pain started initially in his back and was of great severity. He vomited three times and felt dizzy at the onset of the pain. In the past, he has suffered from repeated right-sided pneumothoraces, requiring a pleurodesis 2 years ago. He has also had a number of eye problems and was diagnosed last year with a lens dislocation and blue sclerae. He also has mild asthma for which he takes salbutamol and beclometasone inhalers.

On examination he is a tall, thin man who appears unwell, he is sweating, and has a pulse of 120 beats per minute in sinus rhythm. His blood pressure is 121/82 mmHg. He has a right thoracotomy scar. His abdomen is soft but not tender.

INVESTIGATIONS	RESULTS
Serial ECGs	Sinus tachycardia only
Chest X-ray	No focal lung lesion
	Prominent mediastinum
Creatinine kinase	120 (0–200) IU/l
Plasma sodium	135 mmol/l
Plasma potassium	4.8 mmol/l
Plasma urea	3.2 mmol/l
Plasma creatinine	89 μmol/l
Liver function tests	Normal

ECG: electrocardiogram. Figures in parentheses indicate normal ranges.

a) What is the most likely diagnosis?

b) What two diagnostic tests would you do next?

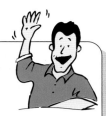

A68   a) **Diagnosis**
Dissecting thoracic aortic aneurysm secondary to
Marfan's syndrome

b) **Diagnosis**
Check the blood pressure in both arms. Magnetic resonance imaging
(MRI) scan would be superior to a CT chest scan, which is superior
to a transoesophageal echocardiogram, which in turn is superior to
a transthoracic echocardiogram

This patient is a fairly classical case of Marfan's syndrome. He is tall and thin and has experienced a number of well-recognised complications of this condition. Again, it is a case of recognising the syndrome and then the answer is obvious.

Answering the question requires the knowledge of a list that we haven't yet given you – causes of blue sclerae.

CAUSES OF BLUE SCLERAE

Remember the POKEMon craze?

- Pseudoxanthoma elasticum
- Osteogenesis imperfecta
- K(c)ongenital
- Ehlers–Danlos syndrome
- Marfan's syndrome

MARFAN'S SYNDROME

"The only way is up" – this song describes the condition beautifully, in particular the way that the lens dislocates (compare it with homocystinuria in which dislocation occurs downwards). Marfan's syndrome has multiple complications that may appear in the written or clinical parts of the examination:

- lung: repeated pneumothoraces
- cardiac: aortic dissection, aortic regurgitation, mitral valve prolapse, regurgitation
- eyes: 'upward' lens dislocation, blue sclera, retinal detachment.

It has to be said, at this point, that one of the authors (NG) has fond memories of a patient with Marfan's who was seen as his MRCP long case. He failed the case and was given a score of 2 out of 6 because he was unable to tell the examiners what the patient's brother did for a living. One of the examiners was heard to tell another candidate who saw the patient later (as a short case) that this patient's brother bred pigs for valve replacements, and they had been failing candidates earlier that day for not telling them this as part of the social history. You have been warned: take a full social history in the examination.

FOR THE RECORD

EJA Marfan (1858–1942), French paediatrician.

Q69 A 43-year-old woman presents to the endocrinology outpatient clinic with recurrent episodes of dizziness with collapse. She is admitted to the hospital for further investigation. During one of these episodes her blood glucose is noted to be 1 mmol/l. A serum sample is sent with the following results – serum glucose 1.3 mmol/l. She has never suffered from diabetes and nor has any member of her family. She is not on any routine medication. In the past, she was investigated for hypercalcaemia and a parathyroid adenoma was discovered that was successfully resected with no long-term problems.

a) What two investigations would you next perform?

b) What is the relationship between hypoglycaemia and a parathyroid adenoma?

A69

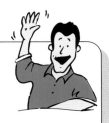

a) **Investigations**
   Insulin C-peptide level
   CT scan of the abdomen looking for an insulinoma

b) **Hypoglycaemia and parathyroid adenoma**
   Multiple endocrine neoplasia (MEN) type I

This patient is under investigation for a cause of her dizziness. Clearly the patient has become hypoglycaemic. The important part of this case is to recognise the link between hypoglycaemia and her pituitary adenoma.

MEN TYPE I (THE 3 Ps) – WERNER'S SYNDROME

- Parathyroid adenoma
- Pancreatic adenoma: insulinoma, Zollinger–Ellison syndrome/gastrinoma and glucagonoma, Cushing's syndrome, and carcinoids are also recognised
- Pituitary tumour

Note: glucagonoma is an islet α-cell-derived pancreatic tumour. The clinical features include:
- necrolytic erythema migrans
- diabetes mellitus
- weight loss
- anaemia
- cheilitis
- stomatitis
- thromboembolism
- gastrointestinal disturbances
- neuropsychiatric disturbances

Glucagon, liver disease, aberrant fatty acids, and zinc deficiency states may also contribute to the pathogenesis of the eruption in some cases – hence the zinc treatment. It is often caught late and is treated with cytotoxic drugs and palliative care.

MEN TYPE II SYNDROMES

These are characterised by their predisposition to medullary thyroid carcinomas, which are seen in 70%–80% of cases, and phaeochromocytomas (seen in 60% of cases).

MEN TYPE IIA (SIPPLE'S SYNDROME)

- Phaeochromocytoma
- Medullary cancer of the thyroid
- Parathyroid hyperplasia
- Hirschsprung's disease

MEN TYPE IIB

- Phaeochromocytoma
- Medullary cancer of the thyroid plus skin (neuromas, pigmentation) plus marfanoid habitus plus intestinal ganglioneuromatosis

TIP

It is important to note that in the MRCP examination, if hypoglycaemia occurs in a healthcare professional, then the examiners may be thinking of insulin or sulphonylurea self-administration. In the latter, the C-peptide level will also be raised, as in insulinoma. Thus, a measure of urinary sulphonylurea must be performed.

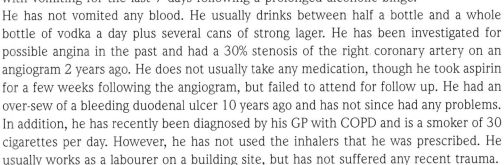

Q70 A 56-year-old man presents with a 3-hour history of central crushing chest pain associated with sweating, nausea, and vomiting. He admits to being unwell, with vomiting for the last 7 days following a prolonged alcoholic binge. He has not vomited any blood. He usually drinks between half a bottle and a whole bottle of vodka a day plus several cans of strong lager. He has been investigated for possible angina in the past and had a 30% stenosis of the right coronary artery on an angiogram 2 years ago. He does not usually take any medication, though he took aspirin for a few weeks following the angiogram, but failed to attend for follow up. He had an over-sew of a bleeding duodenal ulcer 10 years ago and has not since had any problems. In addition, he has recently been diagnosed by his GP with COPD and is a smoker of 30 cigarettes per day. However, he has not used the inhalers that he was prescribed. He usually works as a labourer on a building site, but has not suffered any recent trauma.

On examination he appears unwell, has tachycardia with a pulse of 110 beats/min. His blood pressure is 122/80 mm Hg and he has pyrexia with a temperature of 38.3°C. He also has surgical emphysema in the right supraclavicular fossa and stigmata of chronic liver disease, including a left Dupuytren's contracture, palmar erythema, and multiple spider naevi on his anterior chest wall. He is cardiovascularly stable and has no murmurs. He has a respiratory rate of 20 breaths/min with an oxygen saturation of 91%.

INVESTIGATIONS	RESULTS
Haemoglobin	12.6 g/dl
Mean corpuscular volume	101 fl
White cell count	14.2 x 10⁹/l
Neutrophils	12.8 x 10⁹/l
Platelets	62 x 10⁹/l
Plasma sodium	131 mmol/l
Plasma potassium	3.2 mmol/l
Plasma urea	3.1 mmol/l
Plasma creatinine	93 μmol/l
Serum aspartate aminotransferase	65 (5–15) IU/l
Serum alanine aminotransferase	32 (5–15) IU/l
Serum alkaline phosphatase	195 IU/l
Serum albumin	32 g/l
Serum creatinine kinase	65 (0–190) IU/l
Clotting INR	1.2
ECG	Sinus tachycardia, no evidence of acute ischaemia

ECG: electrocardiogram; INR: international normalised ratio. Figures in parentheses indicate normal ranges.

a) What is the most likely diagnosis?

b) What test will confirm the diagnosis?

ANSWERS TO JIGSAW PUZZLE (see page 240)

	A	C	R	O	M	E	G	A	L	Y	
	R	E	F	S	U	M	S				
T	H	A	L	A	S	S	A	E	M	I	A
	F	R	I	E	D	R	E	I	C	H	S
				A	L	P	O	R	T	S	

Acromegaly and Thalassaemia are causes of angioid retinal streaks.

This initially appears to be a complex question in which there are a lot of leads. However, as is often the case in the MRCP examination, there is a give-away clue. Again, this is a case of spot the clue and the diagnosis is obvious. In this case, the fact that the patient has surgical emphysema and has had prolonged vomiting should quickly lead you to the diagnosis of oesophageal perforation (Boerhaave's syndrome).

A70

a) **Diagnosis**
   Oesophageal perforation (Boerhaave's syndrome) secondary to recurrent vomiting

b) **Test**
   A chest X-ray. In this case it showed mediastinal air. A Gastrografin swallow may also confirm the diagnosis

BOERHAAVE'S SYNDROME

Hermann Boerhaave (1668–1738) was a Dutch physician who was the first to describe oesophageal perforation in a Dutch seaman who presented to him with central chest pain and rapidly died. At autopsy, an oesophageal perforation was diagnosed with the patient's gastric contents within the mediastinum (or so the story goes).

An alternative theory is that all the above is bulls**t and in fact he just decided to have a syndrome named after him, which was a popular pasttime during this era. As many of you are aware, a lot of physical signs have eponymous names.

Q71 An 80-year-old man presents to an Accident and Emergency Department with erythroderma. The only history that was available was from his elderly wife, who was clearly upset and attributed his acute illness to the GP who had given the patient amoxycillin for his third chest infection of the year. Although the patient had suggested he was allergic to penicillin, he had received, against the wishes of his wife, the drug for the first and third infections and a macrolide for the second infection. The wife also felt upset that her husband had recently been given the diagnosis of bronchiectasis. He had also recently suffered from cellulitis, for which he had been given clindamycin.

On examination, the patient has an exfoliative dermatitis with scaling erythematous dermatitis involving 90% or more of the surface area. He was confused and scratching himself uncontrollably. He also had periorbital inflammation, splenomegaly, and retromandibular lymphadenopathy.

Investigations	Results
Haemoglobin	12.6 g/dl
White cell count	35.8 x 10⁹/l
Neutrophils	12.8 x 10⁹/l
Platelets	62 x 10⁹/l
Plasma sodium	131 mmol/l
Plasma potassium	3.2 mmol/l
Plasma urea	15.0 mmol/l
Plasma creatinine	300 μmol/l
Serum aspartate aminotransferase	12 (5–15) IU/l
Serum alanine aminotransferase	12 (5–15) IU/l
Serum alkaline phosphatase	195 IU/l
Serum albumin	20 g/l
Creatinine kinase	300 (0–190) IU/l
Clotting INR	1.0

INR: international normalised ratio. Figures in parentheses indicate normal ranges.

a) What is the cause of this man's acute illness?

This question once again gives you the diagnosis of erythroderma and asks you for the cause. Despite the obvious red herring of the drug-induced erythroderma (who said the examiners were subtle!), clearly the patient has had cellulitis, bronchiectasis, and recurrent pneumonias – he must be immunocompromised. Furthermore, he has splenomegaly and lymphadenopathy. Thus, he must have chronic lymphocytic leukaemia (CLL).

CLL is a clonal proliferation of mature lymphocytes, normally B-cells, with accumulation in the blood, bone marrow, lymph nodes, and the spleen. It is the most common form of leukaemia in adults, predominantly affecting the elderly (mean age 64 years). Its pathogenesis is thought to be linked to abnormal tumour suppressor genes, such as BCL-1 and oncogene C-MYC. Lymphocyte counts are greater than 10,000. Cells can be identified by their cell surface markers: CD19, CD20, and CD5 (note, CD stands for cluster of differentiation). Clinically, patients are often identified incidentally with an indolent lymphocytosis. Lymphadenopathy, organomegaly, and bone marrow involvement with pancytopenia may also be present. Immunological complications include immunoparesis due to depressed immunoglobulin levels, which result in recurrent respiratory and other infections and bronchiectasis. Other immunological phenomena include direct Coombs test-positive haemolytic anaemia and immune thrombocytopenia/neutropenia. CLL can also transform into a number of haematological tumours – the most feared of which is large cell lymphoma. Patients also get homme rouge, which is a form of erythroderma. Please don't be caught out– they have warm haemolytic anaemia (i.e. evidence of haemolysis at room temperature), but *also* have cryoglobulins.

The overall 5-year survival is approximately 60%, but depends on the stage of disease, serum levels of β2-microglobulin, lactate dehydrogenase, CD23 (remember, CD stands for cluster of differentiation), and cytogenetic abnormalities, such as deletions in chromosome 11q and somatic mutations in the immunoglobulin heavy-chain genes. Antileukaemic therapy includes chlorambucil and fludarabine, a purine analogue, steroids, and monoclonal antibodies. Also note the need for antimicrobial therapy.

Rai staging system for CLL

Stage 0	Isolated lymphocytosis ($>15,000/mm^3$)
Stage I	Lymphocytosis with lymphadenopathy
Stage II	Lymphocytosis with splenomegaly
Stage III	Lymphocytosis with anaemia (haemoglobin <11 g/dl)
Stage IV	Lymphocytosis and thrombocytopenia ($<100,000/mm^3$)

Causes of erythroderma

Dermatoses	Atopic dermatitis, candidiasis, contact dermatitis, dermatophytosis (e.g. tinea), ichthyosis, lichen planus, mastocytosis, nummular eczema, pemphigus, photosensitive eczema, pityriasis, psoriasis, Reiter's syndrome, scabies, seborrhoeic dermatitis, and staphylococcal scalded skin syndrome
Autoimmune	SLE
Malignancies	T-cell lymphomas and other lymphomas, leukaemias, and internal visceral malignancies
Drugs	Many!
Miscellaneous	Hepatitis, HIV, congenital immunodeficiency syndromes (Omenn's syndrome), and graft versus host disease

Erythroderma with blood redistribution to the integumentary surface and exfoliation is reminiscent of severe burns. The catabolic state coupled with severe block of hepatic albumin synthesis and surface loss may lead to oedema. The large open wounds may result in sepsis and must be treated with broad-spectrum antibiotics. High-output cardiac failure may result from the massive redistribution of blood to the skin. Management requires close haemodynamic monitoring with covering of wounds to prevent hypothermia and sepsis. Perhaps the most important aspect of treatment is total body coverage with emollients, together with antihistamines for pruritus. Recently, evidence has accumulated for the use of systemic immunosuppression with corticosteroids and cyclosporin.

12

MORE ON EPONYMOUS
CONDITIONS IN THE
MRCP EXAMINATION

To finish our quick trawl through the MRCP examination, here is a list of some of the eponymous syndromes that may appear in the MRCP examination. We have also given a brief line on what these eminent doctors actually did. Be prepared to be shocked by the infamous Dr Reiter!!!

BERNARD–SOULIER SYNDROME

- congenital condition with large platelets associated with a prolongation of the bleeding time
- thrombocytopenia
- due to a specific lack of glycoprotein 1b

Jean Bernard (born 1907), French physician; Jean Pierre Soulier (born 1915), French haematologist

BROWN-SÉQUARD'S SYNDROME

- hemisection of the spinal cord
- contralateral loss of pain and temperature (spinothalamic tracts)
- ipsilateral flaccid paralysis (corticospinal tracts) and loss of touch, conscious proprioception, and vibration (dorsal columns)

Charles Brown-Séquard (1817–1894), French physiologist and neurologist

CHAGAS' DISEASE

- caused by *Trypanosoma cruzi*
- acute: fevers, rash, and meningisms
- chronic: megaoesophagus and cardiomegaly

Carlos Chagas (1879–1934), Brazilian physician

CHÉDIAK–HIGASHI SYNDROME

- neutrophil granule abnormality
- albinism, recurrent bacterial infections

Moisés Chédiak, (born 1903), Cuban physician; Otokata Higashi, 20th Century Japanese paediatrician

CHRISTMAS DISEASE

- sex-linked factor IX deficiency

Christmas: a patient with this disease. Not actually named after Santa Claus.

DARIER'S DISEASE

- pseudoxanthoma elasticum
- keratosis

Jean Darier (1856–1938), French dermatologist

DRESSLER'S SYNDROME

- pericardial or pleural chest pain 4–6 weeks post myocardial infarction or cardiac surgery
- may have pleural/pericardial effusion
- associated with the presence of anticardiolipin antibodies
- may present with associated systemic symptoms

William Dressler (1890–1969), US physician

EATON–LAMBERT SYNDROME

- myasthenic syndrome
- associated with lung cancer

Lee Eaton (1905–1958), US neurologist; Edward Lambert (born 1915), US neurologist

Ehlers–Danlos syndrome

- collagen disorder
- hyperextensibility
- thin elastic skin
- repeated pneumothoraces
- aortic dissection and aortic regurgitation
- mitral valve prolapse

Edward Ehlers (1863–1937), Danish dermatologist; Henri Danlos (1844–1912), French dermatologist

Fanconi's anaemia

- congenital aplastic anaemia
- multiple skeletal abnormalities
- increased risk of leukaemia

Guido Fanconi (1892–1979), Swiss paediatrician

Friedreich's ataxia

- high arched palate
- cerebellar signs
- cardiomyopathy
- dementia
- diabetes
- optic atrophy

Nikolaus Friedreich (1825–1882), German neurologist

Froin's syndrome

- spinal block
- very raised cerebrospinal fluid (CSF) protein

Georges Froin (1874–1932), French neurologist

Gaucher's disease

- defect of β-glucocerebrosidase
- marked hepatosplenomegaly
- pancytopenia

Philippe Gaucher (1854–1918), French physician

Guillain–Barré syndrome

- post-viral polyneuropathy
- ascending motor neuropathy
- high CSF protein

Georges Guillain (1876–1961), French neurologist; Jean Barré (1880–1967), French neurologist

Heerfordt's syndrome

- seen in patients with sarcoidosis
- triad of parotid and lacrimal swelling with uveitis
- may be associated with systemic features

Christian Heerfordt (1871–1953), Danish ophthalmologist

KAWASAKI'S SYNDROME

- most common childhood vasculitis
- unknown aetiology
- systemic illness with conjunctivitis, lymphadenopathy, rash
- 25% develop coronary artery aneurysms
- treated with intravenous gamma globulin

Tomisaku Kawasaki, 20th Century Japanese paediatrician

PRINZMETAL'S ANGINA

- coronary artery spasm
- associated with transient ST elevation

Myron Prinzmetal (1908–1987), US cardiologist

REITER'S SYNDROME

- an old MRCP examination favourite
- keratoderma blenorrhagica (looks like psoriasis on palms and feet)
- genital ulceration and conjunctivitis
- seronegative arthritis
- balanitis circinata
- human leucocyte antigen (HLA) B27 associated
- follows sexually transmitted diseases or enteric infections

Hans Reiter (1881–1969), German bacteriologist. His stance was tainted over the years: he joined Hitler before the Second World War as a physician and remained a staunch supporter throughout the course of the war.

SHY–DRAGER SYNDROME

- autonomic neuropathy
- Parkinsonism

George Milton Shy (1919–1967), US neurologist; Glenn Drager (1917–1967), US neurologist

WALDENSTRÖM'S MACROGLOBULINAEMIA

- often appears in the MRCP examination as a differential diagnosis for myeloma
- patients are not anaemic, and do not have immunosuppression
- usually characterised by a monoclonal increase in IgM

Jan Waldenström (1906–1996), Swedish physician

WEIL'S DISEASE

- spread by contact with rat urine
- in the MRCP examination, it may occur in laboratory workers
- caused by leptospirosis icterohaemorrhagica
- may present with jaundice, fever, oliguria, and haemorrhage

Adolf Weil (1848–1916), German physician

13

THOSE INFAMOUS LISTS AGAIN

A SUMMARY OF **MRCP** EXAMINATION LISTS

1. The strategy

Polyarthralgia

- rheumatoid arthritis (RA), Still's disease
- Henoch–Schönlein purpura
- pseudogout
- systemic lupus erythematosus (SLE)
- infectious: parvovirus, tuberculosis (TB), rubella, varicella zoster virus (VZV), Lyme disease
- familial Mediterranean fever
- Behçet's syndrome
- chronic active hepatitis
- ulcerative colitis/Crohn's disease
- Whipple's disease
- sarcoidosis
- sickle cell disease

2. Nervous ticks on the list: the neurological MRCP lists

Optic atrophy

- congenital Friedreich's ataxia, Leber's optic atrophy, Wolfram's syndrome (DIDMOAD – diabetes insipidus, diabetes mellitus, optic atrophy, deafness)
- papilloedema (longstanding)
- pressure (e.g. compression by tumour and glaucoma)
- poisons (quinine overdose, tobacco amblyopia, wood alcohol)
- Paget's disease
- pernicious anaemia and poor diet (vitamin B_{12} deficiency)
- pulselessness (retinal artery ischaemia)
- syphilis
- multiple sclerosis (MS)

Papilloedema

- benign intracranial pressure
- malignant hypertension
- mass lesions in or around the brain
- hypercapnia
- central retinal vein, or cavernous sinus, or sagital vein thrombosis
- vitamin A toxicity
- lead poisoning and optic neuritis

THIRD NERVE PALSY

- diabetes
- vasculitis: systemic lupus erythematosus (SLE); rheumatoid arthritis (RA); polyarteritis nodosa (PAN)
- malignancy
- compression
- midbrain amyloidosis
- posterior communicating artery aneurysm
- multiple sclerosis (MS)
- cerebrovascular accident (CVA) of midbrain causing Weber's syndrome
- transient and repetitive paroxysmal third nerve palsies can occur with migraines

ANGIOID RETINAL STREAKS

- Paget's disease
- sickle cell anaemia
- Ehlers–Danlos syndrome
- pseudoxanthoma elasticum
- thalassaemia
- acromegaly

CHOROIDORETINITIS

- sarcoidosis
- syphilis
- tuberculosis (TB)
- cytomegalovirus (CMV)
- toxoplasmosis
- toxocariasis

RETINITIS PIGMENTOSA

- hereditary ataxias, such as Friedreich's ataxia
- Refsum's syndrome
- Lawrence–Moon–Biedl syndrome
- Alport's syndrome
- Kearns–Sayre syndrome

CEREBELLAR SYNDROMES: FAT CAT SCAN FOR MS:

- Friedreich's ataxia
- Alcohol
- Tumours
  primary: cerebellar haemangioblastomas
  secondary: especially lung cancer as a paraneoplastic syndrome
- Congenital: ataxia telangiectasia, Arnold–Chiari malformations
- Strokes
- Multiple Sclerosis (MS)

SPASTIC PARAPARESIS

- transverse myelitis complicating a viral infection, multiple sclerosis (MS), or a paraneoplastic syndrome
- sudden vascular occlusion
- tropical spastic paraparesis

ABSENT ANKLE JERKS, EXTENSOR PLANTARS

- syringomyelia
- taboparesis (syphilis)
- Friedreich's ataxia
- cervical spondylosis, peripheral neuropathy
- motor neurone disease
- subacute combined degeneration of the cord

CEREBROSPINAL FLUID (CSF) LYMPHOCYTOSIS

- viral or tuberculous meningitis
- encephalitis
- tumour
- cerebral abscess
- cerebral lymphoproliferative disease
- partially treated bacterial meningitis
- Whipple's disease
- multiple sclerosis (MS)
- systemic lupus erythematosus (SLE)
- Behçet's syndrome
- sarcoidosis

CEREBROSPINAL FLUID (CSF) PROTEIN (RAISED) WITH NORMAL CSF CELLS

- Guillain–Barré syndrome
- lead poisoning
- cord compression
- spinal block (Froin's syndrome)
- cord malignant deposits
- subacute sclerosing panencephalitis
- syphilis

PERIPHERAL POLYNEUROPATHY

- congenital: Friedreich's ataxia, Refsum's disease, Charcot–Marie–Tooth disease
- three dejected: alcoholics due to alcohol; vitamin B_1, B_6, and B_{12} deficiencies; isoniazid for tuberculosis (TB)
- two infected: leprosy, Guillain–Barré syndrome
- two injected: cancer-associated paraneoplasia, or its treatment, such as vincristine and isoniazid; diabetics
- one connected: connective tissue disease, such as: rheumatoid arthritis (RA), systemic lupus erythematosus (SLE), polyarteritis nodosum (PAN)
- sarcoidosis suspected
- hypothyroid

MOTOR NEUROPATHY (ALONE)

- diabetic amyotrophy
- diphtheria
- porphyria (acute intermittent)
- polymyositis
- lead poisoning
- Guillain–Barré syndrome
- cancer-associated paraneoplasia

MONONEURITIS MULTIPLEX

- diabetes mellitus
- leprosy
- connective tissue diseases (polyarteritis nodosum [PAN], systemic lupus erythematosus [SLE], rheumatoid arthritis [RA], giant cell arteritis)
- sarcoidosis
- malignancy
- amyloidosis
- neurofibromatosis
- HIV/AIDS
- Churg–Strauss syndrome

CARPAL TUNNEL SYNDROME

- gout
- tuberculosis (TB)
- pregnancy/oral contraceptive pill
- rheumatoid arthritis (RA)
- renal disease
- acromegaly
- amyloidosis
- myxoedema

3. PANTS: RESPIRATORY MRCP LISTS

PLEURAL EFFUSION

- transudates: congestive heart failure, renal failure, nephrotic syndrome, liver failure, hypoalbuminaemia, peritoneal dialysis, protein-losing enteropathy
- exudates: lung cancer, infection, tuberculosis (TB), vasculitic diseases, yellow nail syndrome, mesothelioma, pulmonary embolism (PE), uraemia, lymphoma, Meig's syndrome, Dressler's syndrome, subphrenic abscess, pancreatitis, hypothyroidism, connective tissue diseases (systemic lupus erythematosis [SLE], rheumatoid arthritis [RA])

Lung fibrosis

- tuberculosis (TB)
- drugs: amiodarone, bleomycin, and busulphan, etc.
- pneumoconioses: silicosis, asbestosis
- acute rheumatic disease (rheumatoid arthritis [RA], systemic lupus erythematosus [SLE], etc.)
- radiation
- sarcoidosis
- hypersensitivty pneumonitis (pigeon breeders' lung, etc.)
- paraquat
- pulmonary haemosiderosis
- histiocytosis X

Remember: Pigeon CRA³PS: cryptogenic fibrosing alveolitis, radiation, amiodarone, (extrinsic) allergic alveolitis, pigeon breeders' lung, sarcoidosis

Cavitation on a chest X-ray

- cancers (particularly squamous cell)
- tuberculosis (TB)
- Wegener's granulomatosis
- rheumatoid nodules, progressive massive fibrosis
- pulmonary embolism (PE)
- histoplasmosis, coccidioidomycosis, aspergillosis
- abscesses (think *Staphylococcus*, *Klebsiella*, amoebiasis, aspiration)

Bronchopulmonary eosinophilia

- adult asthma
- allergic bronchopulmonary aspergillosis
- polyarteritis nodosum (PAN)
- Churg–Strauss syndrome
- Löffler's syndrome
- drugs
- tropical (ascariasis, ankylostomiasis, toxocariasis, strongyloidiasis, filariasis)

Single well-rounded large opacity on a chest X-ray

- neoplasms: primary malignant or metastases; hamartomas
- infections: bacterial, abscesses; tuberculoma; fungal, mycetoma; parasites, hydatid cyst
- vascular: arteriovenous malformations
- haematoma: post-traumatic

Multiple well-rounded large opacity on a chest X-ray

- sarcoidosis
- metastases
- hydatid cysts
- abscesses
- septic emboli

Multiple small (<5 mm) opacities on a chest X-ray
- miliary tuberculosis (TB)
- sarcoidosis
- pneumoconioses
- interstitial fibrosis
- extrinsic allergic alveolitis

Localised radiolucencies
- cavitation in an abscess/carcinoma/tuberculosis (TB)
- bullae
- pneumatoceles (think of cystic fibrosis)
- cystic bronchiectasis

Bilateral hilar lymphadenopathy
- sarcoidosis
- tuberculosis (TB)
- lymphomas
- cancers
- others: cystic fibrosis, Churg–Strauss syndrome, HIV, extrinsic alveolitis, phenytoin treatment, pneumoconioses (especially berylliosis)

Bronchiectasis (TACKY HI²P)
- post tuberculosis (TB)
- aspergillosis
- cystic fibrosis/bronchial compression
- kartagener's syndrome (dysmotile cilia with situs inversus and infertility)
- yellow nail syndrome
- hypogammaglobulinaemia
- idiopathic
- inhalation of foreign body
- post-childhood infection (whooping cough/pertussis, measles)

KCO-low (transfer coefficient of carbon monoxide)
- emphysema
- pulmonary emboli
- pulmonary fibrosis
- ageing
- pulmonary oedema
- low cardiac output states

KCO-high (transfer coefficient of carbon monoxide)
- asthma (although KCO can also be normal)
- pulmonary haemorrhage (Wegener's granulomatosis, Goodpasture's syndrome)
- left-to-right cardiac shunting
- polycythaemia

EOSINOPHILIA

- skins: rheumatoid arthritis with cutaneous manifestations, dermatitis herpetiformis, scabies, eczema

- immune: asthma, atopy, any drug reactions

- neoplastic: lymphomas, acute lymphoblastic leukaemia (ALL), 'all' solid malignancies

- pulmonary eosinophilia

- infective: worms (tapeworm, hookworm, *Filaria*), Whipple's disease, schistosomiasis/other parasites

4. METABOLLOCKS: THE METABOLIC MRCP LISTS

HYPERCALCAEMIA

- excess parathyroid hormone (PTH): primary and tertiary hyperparathyroidism, ectopic PTH (e.g. from oat cell carcinoma of the lung), multiple endocrine neoplasias (MEN) I/II

- vitamin D toxicity

- high hormone levels: Cushing's disease, oestrogen excess, acromegaly, thyrotoxicosis

- metastatic malignancy: the five 'b's: bronchus, breast, byroid, brostate, bidney

- myeloma and lymphoma

- sarcoidosis (phosphate often normal)

- tuberculosis (TB)

- leprosy

- others: milk-alkali syndrome, iatrogenic, idiopathic infantile (supravalvular aortic stenosis, elfin facies), histoplasmosis, coccidioidomycosis, and Wegener's granulomatosis

HYPOCALCAEMIA

- hypoparathyroidism and parathyroid gland excision: pseudohypoparathyroidism

- low vitamin D levels

- malabsorption syndromes

- chronic renal failure

- acute pancreatitis (calcium sequestered as 'soaps')

- rhabdomyolysis

SYNDROME OF INAPPROPRIATE ANTIDIURETIC HORMONE SECRETION (SIADH)

- chest: infections (abscess, effusions, pneumonia, tuberculosis [TB]), tumours (small cell carcinoma especially)

- cerebral: infections (abscess, meningitis, TB); tumours

- drugs: carbamazepine, chlorpropamide, clofibrate, antipsychotic drugs, nonsteroidal anti-inflammatory drugs (NSAIDs)

- cancers: pancreas

- pleural effusions

- pancreatitis

- porphyria

DIABETES INSIPIDUS

- low production: posterior pituitary damage: hypothalamic damage, craniopharyngioma, pituitary stalk damage (e.g. Sheehan's syndrome of pituitary stalk infarction complicating post-partum haemorrhagic shock), pituitary tumours, basal meningitis (particularly tuberculous meningitis), sarcoidosis
- resistance to action: drugs: lithium, or amphotericin therapy

                                electrolytes: prolonged hypercalcaemia or hyponatraemia

                                inherited: nephrogenic diabetes insipidus (X-linked)

HYPOKALAEMIC ALKALOSIS

- steroids: Conn's syndrome, Cushing's disease, corticosteroid treatment, phaeochromocytomas, liquorice, carbenoxolone
- gastrointestinal: vomiting
- villous adenoma
- laxatives
- diuretics: thiazides

HYPOKALAEMIC ACIDOSIS

- partially treated diabetic ketoacidosis
- acetazolamide
- renal tubular acidosis (type I = proximal, type II = distal)
- diarrhoea plus hypovolaemic shock
- enteric (ureterosigmoidostomy or biliary/pancreatic fistula leading to bicarbonate loss: vipoma with MEN I)

RESPIRATORY ACIDOSIS

- respiratory depression: raised intracranial pressure, drugs such as opioids and barbiturates, and overdoses
- neuromuscular disease: neuropathy (such as Guillain–Barré syndrome and motor neurone disease), myopathy
- skeletal disease (ankylosing spondylitis is also a catch)
- chronic obstructive pulmonary disease (COPD)

RESPIRATORY ALKALOSIS

- pulmonary embolism
- early stages of salicylate overdose
- hysterical hyperventilation
- any cause of a metabolic acidosis

METABOLIC ACIDOSIS WITH HIGH ANION GAP

- diabetic ketoacidosis
- lactic acidosis type A (tissue hypoxia): circulatory shock (sepsis, cardiogenic, left ventricular failure [LVF], bleeds, severe anaemia)
- lactic acidosis type B (no tissue hypoxia): acute hepatic failure, renal failure (acute and chronic), leukaemias, biguanides (metformin, phenformin)
- poisoning with acids: salicylates, methanol, ethanol

Metabolic acidosis with normal anion gap

- renal tubular acidosis
- severe diarrhoea (remember villous adenomata, where potassium can be lost in quantity!)
- carbonic anhydrase inhibitors (cause potassium and bicarbonate loss)

Metabolic alkalosis

- acid loss: potassium loss, chloride depletion, pyloric stenosis, hyperaldosteronism
- increased alkali: forced alkaline diuresis, excess alkali in chronic renal failure

Rhabdomyolysis

- trauma: ischaemic muscle damage, bullet wounds, road traffic accidents, compartment syndrome
- severe exertion: paratroopers, prolonged epileptic fits
- alcoholics: via seizures, prolonged immobility, hypophosphataemia
- snake bites
- drug intoxication: cocaine, ecstasy

Renal tubular acidosis type I

- idiopathic
- congenital
- secondary: rheumatoid arthritis (RA), systmatic lupus erythematosus (SLE), Sjögren's syndrome, cirrhosis, sickle cell anaemia, myeloma
- drug-induced: ifosfamide, amphotericin, lithium

Renal tubular acidosis type II

- idiopathic
- congenital: Wilson's disease, cystinosis, galactosaemia, glycogen storage disease type I
- secondary: heavy metals, amyloidosis, paroxysmal nocturnal haemoglobinuria (PNH)
- drugs: carbonic anhydrase inhibitors, ifosfamide

Urea/creatinine ratio elevated

- too much urea made: huge high protein meal, upper gastrointestinal bleed
- low muscle mass: old age with impaired renal function, bilateral amputee with impaired renal function

Glucose tolerance test: lag storage

- post gastrectomy
- liver failure

Hepatomegaly

- biliary cirrhosis
- copper and iron storage diseases
- infections: viral, amoebae, hydatid, Weil's disease
- polycystic disease
- proliferative: lymphoproliferative, myeloproliferative, myeloma, Waldenström's
- raised venous pressure: Budd–Chiari, congestive renal failure

5. HAVE A HEART: THE CARDIOLOGICAL MRCP LISTS

CARDIAC FAILURE AND HEPATOMEGALY

- congestive heart failure (with hepatic engorgement)
- amyloidosis
- lymphoma with cardiac involvement/tamponade
- haemochromatosis
- alcoholic cardiomyopathy

TRICUSPID REGURGITATION

- valve problems: rheumatic heart disease, bacterial endocarditis, congenital heart disease, carcinoid syndrome, myxomatous change
- secondary to elevated pulmonary artery pressures: mitral valve disease, cor pulmonale, primary pulmonary hypertension
- secondary to right ventricular dilatation: right ventricular infarction, any dilated cardiomyopathy

6. SKINNY DIPS: A SELECTION OF DERMATOLOGICAL MRCP LISTS

ERYTHEMA NODOSUM

- sarcoidosis
- tuberculosis (TB)
- inflammatory bowel disease
- infection: streptococcal, histoplasmosis, coccidioidomycosis, North American blastomycosis
- leprosy
- drugs: oral contraceptive pill, sulphonamides, bromides, iodides

ERYTHEMA MULTIFORME

- infection: herpes simplex I/II, *Streptococcus*, *Mycoplasma*, Epstein–Barr virus (EBV), varicella zoster virus (VZV), adenovirus, hepatitis B/C viruses, fungi
- drugs: sulphonamides, sulphonylureas, nonsteroidal anti-inflammatory drugs (NSAIDs), anticonvulsants, barbiturates
- systemic lupus erythematosus (SLE)
- malignancy
- sarcoidosis

CLUBBING

- congenital
- cardiac: subacute bacterial endocarditis (SBE), atrial myxoma, congenital cyanotic heart disease
- respiratory: carcinoma of bronchus, bronchiectasis, cystic fibrosis, pulmonary fibrosis, mesothelioma
- gastrointestinal: inflammatory bowel disease, liver cirrhosis, coeliac disease
- endocrine: thyroid acropachy

7. Gastrointestinal tracts: the GI MRCP lists

Pyoderma gangrenosum

- inflammatory bowel disease
- haematological: myeloma, acute myeloblastic leukaemia (AML), polycythaemia rubra vera (PRV), IgA paraproteinaemia
- connective tissue diseases: systemic lupus erythematosus (SLE), rheumatoid arthritis (RA), polyarteritis nodosa (PAN)

Primary biliary cirrhosis: associated conditions

- rheumatoid arthritis (RA)
- CREST syndrome (calcinosis, Raynaud's disease, oesophageal motility disorder, sclerodactyly and telangiectasia)
- systemic sclerosis
- Sjögren's syndrome
- Hashimoto's disease
- coeliac disease
- dermatomyositis
- renal tubular acidosis

Osteomalacia

- lack of vitamin D: poor diet, low sun exposure
- vitamin D malabsorption: post-gastrectomy, small bowel surgery, biliary disease (e.g. primary biliary cirrhosis), coeliac disease
- renal disease: chronic renal failure; vitamin D-resistant rickets (due to reduced renal tubular phosphate reabsorption); all causes of renal tubular acidosis (proximal and distal)
- miscellaneous: phenytoin-induced osteomalacia; sclerosing haemangiomas; hypophosphataemic rickets; end-organ resistance to 1,25 dihydroxy-vitamin D

8. A bloody hell: haematological MRCP lists

Alkaline phosphatase: raised

- biliary obstruction, cholangiocarcinoma, alcoholic liver disease
- pregnancy
- growing children
- Paget's disease
- temporal arteritis
- metastatic bone or liver disease
- vitamin D deficiency

Leucoerythroblastic blood film

- marrow infiltration: metastases
  - malignancies (myeloma, chronic myelocytic [CML], and acute myeloblastic leukaemia [AML])
  - myelofibrosis
  - myeloproliferative (polycythaemia rarely)
  - mycobacteria (tuberculosis [TB])
  - sarcoidosis
  - storage (Gaucher's disease, Niemann–Pick disease)
- switch on: massive sepsis, massive haemorrhage

PANCYTOPENIA

- viral infections
- drug reactions
- thymic tumours
- hypersplenism
- alcohol
- tuberculosis (TB)
- carcinoma and chemotherapy
- leukaemias and lymphomas
- irradiation
- myelofibrosis, multiple myeloma, megaloblastic anaemia, myelodysplasia
- *Brucella*
- systemic lupus erythematosus (SLE)
- sideroblastic anaemia
- paroxysmal nocturnal haemoglobinuria (PNH)
- parvovirus with sickle cell/haemolytic disease
- Fanconi's syndrome
- Felty's syndrome

HYPERSPLENISM

- infections: tuberculosis (TB), *Brucella*, syphilis, malaria, subacute bacterial endocarditis (SBE), kala azar
- haematological: lymphoma, chronic lymphocytic leukaemia (CLL), chronic myeloblastic leukaemia (CML), myelofibrosis, thalassaemia
- connective tissue: rheumatoid arthritis (RA), Still's disease, Felty's syndrome, systemic lupus erythematosus (SLE)
- metabolic: Gaucher's disease, Niemann–Pick disease
- other: congestion, sarcoidosis, idiopathic

NEUTROPENIA

- pancytopenia
- infection: typhoid, typhus, tuberculosis (TB), any type of viral infection, *Brucella*, kala azar, malaria
- endocrine: hypopituitarism, hypothyroidism, hyperthyroidism
- systemic lupus erythematosus (SLE)
- specific drugs: alcohol and alcoholic cirrhosis, thiouracil

THROMBOCYTOPENIA

- immunological: idiopathic thrombocytopenic purpura (ITP)
- haematological: leukaemia, lymphoma
- massive splenomegaly
- rheumatoid arthritis: Felty's syndrome
- marrow suppression: drugs, HIV, marrow infiltrate
- systemic lupus erythematosus (SLE)
- disseminated intravascular coagulation (DIC): septicaemia, massive bleed, acute respiratory distress syndrome, amniotic fluid embolus, malignancy

POLYCYTHAEMIA

- relative: dehydration, Gaisböck's syndrome (stress)
- primary: polycythaemia rubra vera (PRV) (splenomegaly, raised platelets)
- secondary: hypoxia, chronic obstructive pulmonary disease (COPD), altitude, abnormal haemoglobin, sleep apnoea
- excess erythropoietin: cerebellar haemangioma, hepatoma, phaeochromocytoma, hypernephroma, polycystic/transplant kidneys, uterine leiomyomata/fibromata

ERYTHROCYTE SEDIMENTATION RATE (ESR): LOW

- polycythaemia
- afibrinogenaemia
- hypofibrinogenaemia

ERYTHROCYTE SEDIMENTATION RATE (ESR): VERY HIGH

- temporal arteritis
- polymyalgia rheumatica
- systemic lupus erythematosus (SLE)
- multiple myeloma
- carcinoma
- chronic infection

MACROCYTOSIS

- liver disease
- leucoerythroblastosis
- lead poisoning
- cytotoxic chemotherapy
- reticulocytosis
- renal failure
- respiratory failure
- alcohol ingestion
- aplastic anaemia
- azathioprine treatment
- megaloblastic anaemia (vitamin B_{12}/folate deficiency)
- myeloma
- myxoedema
- malaria
- pregnancy
- pellagra
- primary sideroblastic anaemia

MICROANGIOPATHIC HAEMOLYTIC ANAEMIA (MAHA)

- growths: cancers
  foetuses (eclampsia, abruption, intrauterine death, amniotic fluid embolus)
- renal-failure causes: thrombotic thrombocytopenic purpura (TTP)
  haemolytic uraemic syndrome (HUS)
  acute glomerulonephritis
- small vessel damage: disseminated intravascular coagulation (DIC), malignant hypertension, vasculitides, burns, sepsis
- drugs: cytotoxic agents, cyclosporin

HAEMOLYTIC ANAEMIA

Congenital
- membrane defects: hereditary spherocytosis, hereditary elliptocytosis
- haemoglobinopathies: sickle cell anaemia, thalassaemia
- enzyme defects: glucose-6-phosphate dehydrogenase (G6PD) deficiency, pyruvate kinase deficiency

Acquired
- immune: autoimmune – lymphoma, rheumatoid arthritis (RA); drug-induced – methyldopa, penicillin; post transfusion; paroxysmal nocturnal haemoglobinuria (PNH)
- microangiopathic haemolytic anaemia (MAHA)
- disseminated intravascular coagulation (DIC)
- hypersplenism

HEPATOSPLENOMEGALY WITH LYMPHADENOPATHY

- Waldenström's syndrome
- acute lymphoblastic leukaemia (ALL)
- lymphoma
- lymphoproliferative disorders

SPLENOMEGALY

- massive: chronic myelocytic leukaemia (CML), myelofibrosis, malaria, kala azar, Gaucher's disease
- moderate: all massive disease causes, cirrhosis with portal hypertension, leukaemia, haemolysis, myeloproliferative disease
- mild: all the above, infection, lymphoproliferative disease, immunoproliferative disease, *Brucella*, typhoid, tuberculosis (TB), trypanosomiasis, subacute bacterial endocarditis (SBE), viral infections (infectious mononucleosis, hepatitis B), sarcoidosis, amyloidosis, systemic lupus erythematosus (SLE), Felty's syndrome, idiopathic thrombocytopenic purpura (ITP), haemolysis, iron deficiency, pernicious anaemia

LEUCOCYTE ALKALINE PHOSPHATASE (LAP) SCORE, HIGH

- myeloproliferative disorders: polycythaemia rubra vera (PRV), myelofibrosis, Hodgkin's disease
- steroids: Cushing's disease, treatment with steroids, the pill, pregnancy
- Down's syndrome
- hypoproteinaemia

Leucocyte alkaline phosphatase (LAP) score, low:

- chronic myelocytic leukaemia (CML)
- pernicious anaemia
- idiopathic membranous nephropathy (IMN)
- paroxysmal nocturnal haemoglobinuria (PNH)
- rickets
- hypophosphataemia

Granulomata

- sarcoidosis
- tuberculosis (TB) (caseating)
- Langerhans cell histiocytosis
- Wegener's granulomatosis
- Churg–Strauss disease
- fungal and helminthic infections
- hypersensitivity reactions (e.g. dust)
- malignancy: primary or secondary to colon, kidney, germ-cell, bone, prostate, melanoma

9. Taking the P**s: renal MRCP lists

Nephrotic syndrome

- glomerulonephritis
- subacute bacterial endocarditis (SBE)
- systemic lupus erythematosus (SLE)
- rheumatoid arthritis (RA) treatment (gold and penicillamine)
- polyarteritis nodosum (PAN)
- malaria (*Plasmodium malariae*)
- amyloidosis
- sickle cell anaemia
- cancer (particularly lymphoma)
- bee stings
- renal vein thrombosis
- nonsteroidal anti-inflammatory drugs (NSAIDs)
- captopril
- interferon-α
- heroin

NEPHROTIC SYNDROME, COMPLICATIONS:

- thrombosis
- hyperlipidaemia
- hyponatraemia
- osteomalacia
- malnutrition
- vitamin B_{12} and iron deficiency
- infection
- immunodeficiency
- Budd–Chiari syndrome

RED CELL CASTS IN THE URINE

- glomerulonephritis
- interstitial nephritis
- accelerated hypertension
- haemolytic uraemic syndrome (HUS)

RETROPERITONEAL FIBROSIS

- drugs: practolol, methysergide therapy
- aortic aneurysm
- lymphoma
- radiation
- idiopathic

10. Sex: the MRCP list of sexual medicine

GALACTORRHOEA

- pregnancy
- excess oestrogens
- hypothalamic/pituitary lesions
- prolactinoma and ectopic prolactin secretion
- bronchogenic carcinoma
- hypernephroma
- antidopaminergic drugs: phenothiazines, butyrophenones, metoclopramide, methyldopa
- hypothyroidism
- chronic renal failure
- polycystic ovaries

11. Mopping up

Recurrent deep venous thrombosis

- thrombophilia: antithrombin III deficiency, protein S/C deficiencies, factor V Leiden mutation
- dysfibrinogenaemia
- factor XII deficiency
- malignancy
- surgery and trauma
- post operative
- drugs: oral contraceptive pill
- hyperhomocystinaemia
- Behçet's syndrome
- antiphospholipid syndrome
- paroxysmal nocturnal haemoglobinuria (PNH)
- nephrotic syndrome

Anterior uveitis

- infectious: cytomegalovirus (CMV), toxoplasmosis, syphilis, tuberculosis (TB)
- neoplastic conditions: lymphomas
- systemic diseases: ankylosing spondylitis, Reiter's syndrome, Behçet's syndrome, sarcoidosis, inflammatory bowel disease (IBD), psoriatic arthropathy, juvenile arthritis, Kawasaki disease
- drug induced: rifabutin

Blue sclera

- congenital
- pseudoxanthoma elasticum
- osteogenesis imperfecta
- Ehlers–Danlos syndrome
- Marfan's syndrome

Oral ulceration: recurrent

- aphthous ulcers
- ulcerative colitis/Crohn's disease
- Behçets disease
- coeliac disease
- other causes of malabsorption
- systemic lupus erythematosus (SLE)
- Reiter's disease
- seronegative arthritis
- pemphigus (and, rarely, pemphigoid)

ALL THE LISTS, IN ALPHABETICAL ORDER:

ABSENT ANKLE JERKS, EXTENSOR PLANTARS

- syringomyelia
- taboparesis (syphilis)
- Friedreich's ataxia
- cervical spondylosis, peripheral neuropathy
- motor neurone disease
- subacute combined degeneration of the cord

ALKALINE PHOSPHATASE, RAISED

- biliary obstruction, cholangiocarcinoma, alcoholic liver disease
- pregnancy
- growing children
- Paget's disease
- temporal arteritis
- metastatic bone or liver disease
- vitamin D deficiency

ANGIOID RETINAL STREAKS

- Paget's disease
- sickle cell anaemia
- Ehlers–Danlos syndrome
- pseudoxanthoma elasticum
- thalassaemia
- acromegaly

ANTERIOR UVEITIS

- infectious: cytomegalovirus (CMV), toxoplasmosis, syphilis, tuberculosis (TB)
- neoplastic conditions: lymphomas
- systemic diseases: ankylosing spondylitis, Reiter's syndrome, Behçet's syndrome, sarcoidosis, inflammatory bowel disease (IBD), psoriatic arthropathy, juvenile arthritis, Kawasaki disease
- drug induced: rifabutin

BILATERAL HILAR LYMPHADENOPATHY

- sarcoidosis
- tuberculosis (TB)
- lymphomas
- cancers
- others: cystic fibrosis, Churg–Strauss syndrome, HIV, extrinsic alveolitis, phenytoin treatment, pneumoconioses (especially berylliosis)

BLUE SCLERA

- congenital
- pseudoxanthoma elasticum
- osteogenesis imperfecta
- Ehlers–Danlos syndrome
- Marfan's syndrome

BRONCHIECTASIS (TACKY HI^{2}P)
- post tuberculosis (TB)
- Aspergillosis
- cystic fibrosis/bronchial compression
- kartagener's syndrome (dysmotile cilia with situs inversus and infertility)
- yellow nail syndrome
- hypogammaglobulinaemia
- idiopathic
- inhalation of foreign body
- post-childhood infection (whooping cough/pertussis, measles)

BRONCHOPULMONARY EOSINOPHILIA
- adult asthma
- allergic bronchopulmonary aspergillosis
- polyarteritis nodosum (PAN)
- Churg–Strauss syndrome
- Löffler's syndrome
- drugs
- tropical (ascariasis, ankylostomiasis, toxocariasis, strongyloidiasis, filariasis)

CARDIAC FAILURE AND HEPATOMEGALY
- congestive heart failure (with hepatic engorgement)
- amyloidosis
- lymphoma with cardiac involvement/tamponade
- haemochromatosis
- alcoholic cardiomyopathy

CARPAL TUNNEL SYNDROME
- gout
- tuberculosis (TB)
- pregnancy/oral contraceptive pill
- rheumatoid arthritis (RA)
- renal disease
- acromegaly
- amyloidosis
- myxoedema

CAVITATION ON A CHEST X-RAY
- cancers (particularly squamous cell)
- tuberculosis (TB)
- Wegener's granulomatosis
- rheumatoid nodules, progressive massive fibrosis
- pulmonary embolism (PE)
- histoplasmosis, coccidioidomycosis, aspergillosis
- abscesses (think *Staphylococcus*, *Klebsiella*, amoebiasis, aspiration)

CEREBELLAR SYNDROMES: FAT CAT SCAN FOR MS:

- Friedreich's ataxia
- Alcohol
- Tumours   primary: cerebellar haemangioblastomas
                 secondary: especially lung cancer as a paraneoplastic syndrome
- Congenital: ataxia telangiectasia, Arnold–Chiari malformations
- Strokes
- Multiple Sclerosis (MS)

CEREBROSPINAL FLUID (CSF) LYMPHOCYTOSIS

- viral or tuberculous meningitis
- encephalitis
- tumour
- cerebral abscess
- cerebral lymphoproliferative disease
- partially treated bacterial meningitis
- Whipple's disease
- multiple sclerosis (MS)
- systemic lupus erythematosus (SLE)
- Behçet's syndrome
- sarcoidosis

CEREBROSPINAL FLUID (CSF) PROTEIN (RAISED) WITH NORMAL CSF CELLS

- Guillain–Barré syndrome
- lead poisoning
- cord compression
- spinal block (Froin's syndrome)
- cord malignant deposits
- subacute sclerosing panencephalitis
- syphilis

CHOROIDORETINITIS

- sarcoidosis
- syphilis
- tuberculosis (TB)
- cytomegalovirus (CMV)
- toxoplasmosis
- toxocariasis

CLUBBING

- congenital
- cardiac: subacute bacterial endocarditis (SBE), atrial myxoma, congenital cyanotic heart disease
- respiratory: carcinoma of bronchus, bronchiectasis, cystic fibrosis, pulmonary fibrosis, mesothelioma
- gastrointestinal: inflammatory bowel disease, liver cirrhosis, coeliac disease
- endocrine: thyroid acropachy

Deep venous thrombosis, recurrent

- thrombophilia: antithrombin III deficiency, protein S/C deficiencies, factor V Leiden mutation
- dysfibrinogenaemia
- factor XII deficiency
- malignancy
- surgery and trauma
- post operative
- drugs: oral contraceptive pill
- hyperhomocystinaemia
- Behçet's syndrome
- antiphospholipid syndrome
- paroxysmal nocturnal haemoglobinuria (PNH)
- nephrotic syndrome

Diabetes insipidus

- low production: posterior pituitary damage: hypothalamic damage, craniopharyngioma, pituitary stalk damage (e.g. Sheehan's syndrome of pituitary stalk infarction complicating post-partum haemorrhagic shock), pituitary tumours, basal meningitis (particularly tuberculous meningitis), sarcoidosis
- resistance to action:

drugs:	lithium, or amphotericin therapy
electrolytes:	prolonged hypercalcaemia or hyponatraemia
inherited:	nephrogenic diabetes insipidus (X-linked)

Eosinophilia

- skin: rheumatoid arthritis with cutaneous manifestations, dermatitis herpetiformis, scabies, eczema
- immune: asthma, atopy, any drug reactions
- neoplastic: lymphomas, acute lymphoblastic leukaemia (ALL), 'all' solid malignancies
- pulmonary eosinophilia
- infective: worms (tapeworm, hookworm, Filaria), Whipple's disease, schistosomiasis/other parasites

Erythema multiforme

- infection: herpes simplex I/II, *Streptococcus*, *Mycoplasma*, Epstein–Barr virus (EBV), varicella zoster virus (VZV), adenovirus, hepatitis B/C viruses, fungi
- drugs: sulphonamides, sulphonylureas, nonsteroidal anti-inflammatory drugs (NSAIDs), anticonvulsants, barbiturates
- systemic lupus erythematosus (SLE)
- malignancy
- sarcoidosis

Erythema nodosum

- sarcoidosis
- tuberculosis (TB)
- inflammatory bowel disease
- infection: streptococcal, histoplasmosis, coccidioidomycosis, North American blastomycosis
- leprosy
- drugs: oral contraceptive pill, sulphonamides, bromides, iodides

Erythrocyte sedimentation rate (ESR), (very) high

- temporal arteritis
- polymyalgia rheumatica
- systemic lupus erythematosus (SLE)
- multiple myeloma
- carcinoma
- chronic infection

ERYTHROCYTE SEDIMENTATION RATE (ESR), LOW

- polycythaemia
- afibrinogenaemia
- hypofibrinogenaemia

GALACTORRHOEA

- pregnancy
- excess oestrogens
- hypothalamic/pituitary lesions
- prolactinoma and ectopic prolactin secretion
- bronchogenic carcinoma
- hypernephroma
- antidopaminergic drugs: phenothiazines, butyrophenones, metoclopramide, methyldopa
- hypothyroidism
- chronic renal failure
- polycystic ovaries

GLUCOSE TOLERANCE TEST: LAG STORAGE

- post gastrectomy
- liver failure

GRANULOMATA

- sarcoidosis
- tuberculosis (TB) (caseating)
- Langerhans cell histiocytosis
- Wegener's granulomatosis
- Churg–Strauss disease
- fungal and helminthic infections
- hypersensitivity reactions (e.g. dust)
- malignancy: primary or secondary to colon, kidney, germ-cell, bone, prostate, melanoma

HAEMOLYTIC ANAEMIA

Congenital

- membrane defects: hereditary spherocytosis, hereditary elliptocytosis
- haemoglobinopathies: sickle cell anaemia, thalassaemia
- enzyme defects: glucose-6-phosphate dehydrogenase (G6PD) deficiency, pyruvate kinase deficiency

Acquired

- immune: autoimmune – lymphoma, rheumatoid arthritis (RA); drug-induced – methyldopa, penicillin; post transfusion; paroxysmal nocturnal haemoglobinuria (PNH)
- microangiopathic haemolytic anaemia (MAHA)
- disseminated intravascular coagulation (DIC)
- hypersplenism

HEPATOMEGALY

- biliary cirrhosis
- copper and iron storage diseases
- infections: viral, amoebae, hydatid, Weil's disease
- polycystic disease
- proliferative: lymphoproliferative, myeloproliferative, myeloma, Waldenström's
- raised venous pressure: Budd–Chiari, congestive renal failure

HEPATOSPLENOMEGALY WITH LYMPHADENOPATHY

- Waldenstrom's syndrome
- acute lymphoblastic leukaemia (ALL)
- lymphoma
- lymphoproliferative disorders

HYPERCALCAEMIA

- excess parathyroid hormone (PTH): primary and tertiary hyperparathyroidism, ectopic PTH (e.g. from oat cell carcinoma of the lung), multiple endocrine neoplasias (MEN) I/II
- vitamin D toxicity
- high hormone levels: Cushing's disease, oestrogen excess, acromegaly, thyrotoxicosis
- metastatic malignancy: the five 'b's: bronchus, breast, byroid, brostate, bidney
- myeloma and lymphoma
- sarcoidosis (phosphate often normal)
- tuberculosis (TB)
- leprosy
- others: milk-alkali syndrome, iatrogenic, idiopathic infantile (supravalvular aortic stenosis, elfin facies), histoplasmosis, coccidioidomycosis, and Wegener's granulomatosis

HYPERSPLENISM

- infections: tuberculosis (TB), *Brucella*, syphilis, malaria, subacute bacterial endocarditis (SBE), kala azar
- haematological: lymphoma, chronic lymphocytic leukaemia (CLL) chronic myeloblastic leukaemia (CML), myelofibrosis, thalassaemia
- connective tissue: rheumatoid arthritis (RA), Still's disease, Felty's syndrome, systemic lupus erythematosus (SLE)
- metabolic: Gaucher's disease, Niemann–Pick disease
- other: congestion, sarcoidosis, idiopathic

HYPOCALCAEMIA

- hypoparathyroidism and parathyroid gland excision: pseudohypoparathyroidism
- low vitamin D levels
- malabsorption syndromes
- chronic renal failure
- acute pancreatitis (calcium sequestered as 'soaps')
- rhabdomyolysis

HYPOKALAEMIC ACIDOSIS WITH NORMAL ANION GAP

- partially treated diabetic ketoacidosis
- acetazolamide
- renal tubular acidosis (type I = proximal, type II = distal)
- diarrhoea plus hypovolaemic shock
- enteric (ureterosigmoidostomy or biliary/pancreatic fistula leading to bicarbonate loss: vipoma with multiple endocrine neoplasia [MEN] I)

HYPOKALAEMIC ALKALOSIS

- steroids: Conn's syndrome, Cushing's disease, corticosteroid treatment, phaeochromocytomas, liquorice, carbenoxolone
- gastrointestinal: vomiting
- villous adenoma
- laxatives
- diuretics: thiazides

KCO-HIGH (transfer coefficient of carbon monoxide)
- asthma (although KCO can also be normal)
- pulmonary haemorrhage (Wegener's granulomatosis, Goodpasture's syndrome)
- left-to-right cardiac shunting
- polycythaemia

KCO-LOW (transfer coefficient of CARBON MONOXIDE)
- emphysema
- pulmonary emboli
- pulmonary fibrosis
- ageing
- pulmonary oedema
- low cardiac output states

LEUCOCYTE ALKALINE PHOSPHATASE (LAP) SCORE, HIGH
- myeloproliferative disorders: polycythaemia rubra vera (PRV), myelofibrosis, Hodgkin's disease
- steroids: Cushing's disease, treatment with steroids, the pill, pregnancy
- Down's syndrome
- hypoproteinaemia

LEUCOCYTE ALKALINE PHOSPHATASE (LAP) SCORE, LOW
- chronic myelocytic leukaemia (CML)
- pernicious anaemia
- idiopathic membranous nephropathy (IMN)
- paroxysmal nocturnal haemoglobinuria (PNH)
- rickets
- hypophosphataemia

LEUCOERYTHROBLASTIC BLOOD FILM
- marrow infiltration: metastases
  malignancies (myeloma, chronic myelocytic [CML], and acute myeloblastic leukaemia [AML])
  myelofibrosis
  myeloproliferative (polycythaemia rarely)
  mycobacteria (tuberculosis [TB])
  sarcoidosis
  storage (Gaucher's disease, Niemann–Pick disease)
- switch on: massive sepsis, massive haemorrhage

LUNG FIBROSIS
- tuberculosis (TB)
- drugs: amiodarone, bleomycin, busulphan, etc.
- pneumoconioses: silicosis, asbestosis
- acute rheumatic disease (rheumatoid arthritits [RA], systematic lupus erythematosus [SLE], etc.)
- radiation
- sarcoidosis
- hypersensitivity pneumonitis (pigeon breeders' lung, etc.)
- paraquat
- pulmonary haemosiderosis
- histiocytosis X

Remember: Pigeon CRA³PS: cryptogenic fibrosing alveolitis, radiation, amiodarone, (extrinsic) allergic alveolitis, pigeon breeders lung', sarcoidosis

MACROCYTOSIS

- liver disease
- leucoerythroblastosis
- lead poisoning
- cytotoxic chemotherapy
- reticulocytosis
- renal failure
- respiratory failure
- alcohol ingestion
- aplastic anaemia
- azathioprine treatment
- megaloblastic anaemia (vitamin B_{12}/folate deficiency)
- myeloma
- myxoedema
- malaria
- pregnancy
- pellagra
- primary sideroblastic anaemia

METABOLIC ACIDOSIS WITH HIGH ANION GAP

- diabetic ketoacidosis
- lactic acidosis type A (tissue hypoxia): circulatory shock (sepsis, cardiogenic, left ventricular failure [LVF], bleeds, severe anaemia)
- lactic acidosis type B (no tissue hypoxia): acute hepatic failure, renal failure (acute and chronic), leukaemias, biguanides (metformin, phenformin)
- poisoning with acids: salicylates, methanol, ethanol

METABOLIC ACIDOSIS WITH NORMAL ANION GAP

- renal tubular acidosis
- severe diarrhoea (remember villous adenomata, where potassium can be lost in quantity!)
- carbonic anhydrase inhibitors (cause potassium and bicarbonate loss)

METABOLIC ALKALOSIS

- acid loss: potassium loss, chloride depletion, pyloric stenosis, hyperaldosteronism
- increased alkali: forced alkaline diuresis, excess alkali in chronic renal failure

MICROANGIOPATHIC HAEMOLYTIC ANAEMIA (MAHA)

growths:	cancers
	foetuses (eclampsia, abruption, intrauterine death, amniotic fluid embolus)
renal-failure causes:	thrombotic thrombocytopenic purpura (TTP)
	haemolytic uraemic syndrome (HUS)
	acute glomerulonephritis
small vessel damage:	disseminated intravascular coagulation (DIC), malignant hypertension, vasculitides, burns, sepsis
drugs:	cytotoxic agents, cyclosporin

MONONEURITIS MULTIPLEX

- diabetes mellitus
- leprosy
- connective tissue diseases (polyarteritis nodosum [PAN], systemic lupus erythematosus [SLE], rheumatoid arthritis [RA], giant cell arteritis)
- sarcoidosis
- malignancy
- amyloidosis
- neurofibromatosis
- HIV/AIDS
- Churg–Strauss syndrome

MOTOR NEUROPATHY (ALONE)

- diabetic amyotrophy
- diphtheria
- porphyria (acute intermittent)
- polymyositis
- lead poisoning
- Guillain–Barré syndrome
- cancer-associated paraneoplasia

NEPHROTIC SYNDROME

- glomerulonephritis
- subacute bacterial endocarditis (SBE)
- systemic lupus erythematosus (SLE)
- rheumatoid arthritis (RA) treatment (gold and penicillamine)
- polyarteritis nodosum (PAN)
- malaria *(Plasmodium malariae)*
- amyloidosis
- sickle cell anaemia
- cancer (particularly lymphoma)
- bee stings
- renal vein thrombosis
- nonsteroidal anti-inflammatory drugs (NSAIDs)
- captopril
- interferon-α
- heroin

Nephrotic syndrome, complications

- thrombosis
- hyperlipidaemia
- hyponatraemia
- osteomalacia
- malnutrition
- vitamin B_{12} and iron deficiency
- infection
- immunodeficiency
- Budd–Chiari syndrome

Neutropenia

- pancytopenia
- infection: typhoid, typhus, tuberculosis (TB), any type of viral infection, *Brucella*, kala azar, malaria
- endocrine: hypopituitarism, hypothyroidism, hyperthyroidism
- systemic lupus erythematosus (SLE)
- specific drugs: alcohol and alcoholic cirrhosis, thiouracil

Opacities on a chest X-ray: multiple, small (<5 mm)

- miliary tuberculosis (TB)
- sarcoidosis
- pneumoconioses
- interstitial fibrosis
- extrinsic allergic alveolitis

Opacity on a chest X-ray: multiple, well-rounded, large

- sarcoidosis
- metastases
- hydatid cysts
- abscesses
- septic emboli

Opacity on a chest X-ray: single, well-rounded, large

- neoplasms: primary malignant or metastases; hamartomas
- infections: bacterial, abscesses; tuberculoma; fungal, mycetoma; parasites, hydatid cyst
- vascular: arteriovenous malformations
- haematoma: post-traumatic

Optic atrophy

- congenital Friedreich's ataxia, Leber's optic atrophy, Wolfram's syndrome (DIDMOAD – diabetes insipidus, diabetes mellitus, optic atrophy, deafness)
- papilloedema (longstanding)
- pressure (e.g. compression by tumour and glaucoma)
- poisons (quinine overdose, tobacco amblyopia, wood alcohol)
- Paget's disease
- pernicious anaemia and poor diet (vitamin B_{12} deficiency)
- pulselessness (retinal artery ischaemia)
- syphilis
- multiple sclerosis (MS)

Oral ulceration: recurrent

- aphthous ulcers
- ulcerative colitis/Crohn's disease
- Behçet's disease
- coeliac disease
- other causes of malabsorption
- systemic lupus erythematosus (SLE)
- Reiter's disease
- seronegative arthritis
- pemphigus (and, rarely, pemphigoid)

OSTEOMALACIA

- lack of vitamin D: poor diet; low sun exposure
- vitamin D malabsorption: post-gastrectomy, small bowel surgery, biliary disease (e.g. primary biliary cirrhosis), coeliac disease
- renal disease: chronic renal failure; vitamin D-resistant rickets (due to reduced renal tubular phosphate reabsorption); all causes of renal tubular acidosis (proximal and distal)
- miscellaneous: phenytoin-induced osteomalacia; sclerosing haemangiomas; hypophosphataemic rickets; end-organ resistance to 1,25 dihydroxy-vitamin D

PANCYTOPENIA

- viral infections
- drug reactions
- thymic tumours
- hypersplenism
- alcohol
- tuberculosis (TB)
- carcinoma and chemotherapy
- leukaemias and lymphomas
- irradiation
- myelofibrosis, multiple myeloma, megaloblastic anaemia, myelodysplasia
- *Brucella*
- systemic lupus erythematosus (SLE)
- sideroblastic anaemia
- paroxymal nocturnal haemoglobinuria (PNH)
- parvovirus with sickle cell/haemolytic disease
- Fanconi's syndrome
- Felty's syndrome

PAPILLOEDEMA

- benign intracranial pressure
- malignant hypertension
- mass lesions in or around the brain
- hypercapnia
- central retinal vein, cavernous sinus, or sagittal vein thrombosis
- hydrocephalus
- vitamin A toxicity
- lead poisoning and optic neuritis

PERIPHERAL POLYNEUROPATHY

- congenital: Friedreich's ataxia, Refsum's disease, Charcot–Marie–Tooth disease
- three dejected: alcoholics due to alcohol; vitamin B_1, B_6, and B_{12} deficiencies; isoniazid for tuberculosis (TB)
- two infected: leprosy, Guillain–Barré syndrome
- two injected: cancer-associated paraneoplasia, or its treatment, such as vincristine and isoniazid; diabetics
- one connected: connective tissue disease, such as rheumatoid arthritis (RA), systemic lupus erythematosus (SLE), polyarteritis nodosum (PAN)
- sarcoidosis suspected
- hypothyroid

PLEURAL EFFUSION

- transudates: congestive heart failure, renal failure, nephrotic syndrome, liver failure, hypoalbuminaemia, peritoneal dialysis, protein-losing enteropathy
- exudates: lung cancer, infection, tuberculosis (TB), vasculitic diseases, yellow nail syndrome, mesothelioma, pulmonary embolism (PE), uraemia, lymphoma, Meig's syndrome, Dressler's syndrome, subphrenic abscess, pancreatitis, hypothyroidism, connective tissue diseases (systemic lupus erythematosis [SLE], rheumatoid arthritis [RA])

POLYARTHRALGIA

- rheumatoid arthritis (RA), Still's disease
- Henoch–Schönlein purpura
- pseudogout
- systemic lupus erythematosus (SLE)
- infectious: parvovirus, tuberculosis (TB), rubella, varicella zoster virus (VZV), Lyme disease
- familial Mediterranean fever
- Behçet's syndrome
- chronic active hepatitis
- ulcerative colitis/Crohn's disease
- Whipple's disease
- sarcoidosis
- sickle cell disease

POLYCYTHAEMIA

- relative: dehydration, Gaisböck's syndrome (stress)
- primary: polycythaemia rubra vera (PRV)
- secondary: hypoxia, chronic obstructive pulmonary disease (COPD), altitude
- excess erythropoietin: cerebellar haemangioma, hepatoma, hypernephroma, uterine leiomyomata/fibromata

PRIMARY BILIARY CIRRHOSIS: ASSOCIATED CONDITIONS

- rheumatoid arthritis (RA)
- CREST syndrome (calcinosis, Raynaud's disease, oesophageal motility disorder, sclerodactyly and telangiectasia
- systemic sclerosis
- Sjögren's syndrome
- Hashimoto's disease
- coeliac disease
- dermatomyositis
- renal tubular acidosis

PYODERMA GANGRENOSUM

- inflammatory bowel disease
- haematological: myeloma, acute myeloblastic leukaemia (AML), polycythaemia rubra vera (PRV), IgA paraproteinaemia
- connective tissue diseases: systemic lupus erythematosus (SLE), rheumatoid arthritis (RA), polyarteritis nodosum (PAN)

RADIOLUCENCIES, LOCALISED

- cavitation in an abscess/carcinoma/tuberculosis (TB)
- bullae
- pneumatoceles (think of cystic fibrosis)
- cystic bronchiectasis

RED CELL CASTS IN THE URINE

- glomerulonephritis
- interstitial nephritis
- accelerated hypertension
- haemolytic uraemic syndrome (HUS)

RENAL TUBULAR ACIDOSIS TYPE I

- idiopathic
- congenital
- secondary: rheumatoid arthritis (RA), systemic lupus erythematosus (SLE), Sjögren's syndrome, cirrhosis, sickle cell anaemia, myeloma
- drug-induced: ifosfamide, amphotericin, lithium

RENAL TUBULAR ACIDOSIS TYPE II

- idiopathic
- congenital: Wilson's disease, cystinosis, galactosaemia, glycogen storage disease type I
- secondary: heavy metals, amyloidosis, paroxysmal nocturnal haemoglobinuria (PNH)
- drugs: carbonic anhydrase inhibitors, ifosfamide

RESPIRATORY ACIDOSIS

- respiratory depression: raised intracranial pressure, drugs such as opioids and barbiturates, and overdoses
- neuromuscular disease: neuropathy (such as Guillain–Barré syndrome and motor neurone disease), myopathy
- skeletal disease (ankylosing spondylitis is also a catch)
- chronic obstructive pulmonary disease (COPD)

RESPIRATORY ALKALOSIS

- pulmonary embolism
- early stages of salicylate overdose
- hysterical hyperventilation
- any cause of a metabolic acidosis

RETINITIS PIGMENTOSA

- hereditary ataxias, such as Friedreich's ataxia
- Refsum's syndrome
- Lawrence–Moon–Biedl syndrome
- Alport's syndrome
- Kearns–Sayre syndrome

RETROPERITONEAL FIBROSIS

- drugs: practolol, methysergide therapy
- aortic aneurysm
- lymphoma
- radiation
- idiopathic

RHABDOMYOLYSIS

- trauma: ischaemic muscle damage, bullet wounds, road traffic accidents, compartment syndrome
- severe exertion: paratroopers, prolonged epileptic fits
- alcoholics: via seizures, prolonged immobility, hypophosphataemia
- snake bites
- drug intoxication: cocaine, ecstasy

SPASTIC PARAPARESIS

- transverse myelitis complicating a viral infection, multiple sclerosis (MS), or a paraneoplastic syndrome
- sudden vascular occlusion
- tropical spastic paraparesis

Splenomegaly

- massive: chronic myelocytic leukaemia (CML), myelofibrosis, malaria, kala azar, Gaucher's disease
- moderate: all massive disease causes, cirrhosis with portal hypertension, leukaemia, haemolysis, myeloproliferative disease
- mild: all the above, infection, lymphoproliferative disease, immunoproliferative disease, *Brucella*, typhoid, tuberculosis (TB), trypanosomiasis, subacute bacterial endocarditis (SBE), viral infections (infectious mononucleosis, hepatitis B), sarcoidosis, amyloidosis,
systemic lupus erythematosus (SLE), Felty's syndrome, immune thrombocytopenic purpura (ITP), haemolysis, iron deficiency, pernicious anaemia

Syndrome of inappropriate antidiuretic hormone secretion (SIADH)

- chest: infections (abscess, effusions, pneumonia, tuberculosis [TB]); tumours (small cell carcinoma especially)
- cerebral: infections (abscess, meningitis, TB), tumours
- drugs: carbamazepine, chlorpropamide, clofibrate, antipsychotic drugs, nonsteroidal anti-inflammatory drugs (NSAIDs)
- cancers: pancreas
- pleural effusions
- pancreatitis
- porphyria

Third nerve palsy

- diabetes
- vasculitis: systemic lupus erythematosus (SLE); rheumatoid arthritis (RA); polyarteritis nodosa (PAN)
- malignancy
- compression
- midbrain amyloidosis
- posterior communicating artery aneurysm
- multiple sclerosis (MS)
- cardiovascular accident (CVA) of midbrain causing Weber's syndrome
- transient and repetitive paroxysmal third nerve palsies can occur with migraines

Thrombocytopaenia

- immunological: idiopathic thrombocytopenic purpura (ITP)
- haematological: leukaemia, lymphoma
- massive splenomegaly
- rheumatoid arthritis: Felty's syndrome
- marrow suppression: drugs, HIV, marrow infiltrate
- systemic lupus erythematosus (SLE)
- disseminated intravascular coagulation (DIC): septicaemia, massive bleed, acute respiratory distress syndrome, amniotic fluid embolus, malignancy

Tricuspid regurgitation

- valve problems: rheumatic heart disease, bacterial endocarditis, congenital heart disease, carcinoid syndrome, myxomatous change
- secondary to elevated pulmonary artery pressures: mitral valve disease, cor pulmonale, primary pulmonary hypertension
- secondary to right ventricular dilatation: right ventricular infarction, any dilated cardiomyopathy

Urea/creatinine ratio elevated

- Too much urea made: huge high protein meal, upper gastrointestinal bleed
- Low muscle mass: old age with impaired renal function, bilateral amputee with impaired renal function